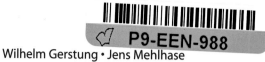

Wilhelm Gerstung • Jens Mehlhase

The Complete Feng Shui Health Handbook

How You Can Protect Yourself Against Harmful Energies and Create Positive Forces for Health and Prosperity

Translated by: Christine M. Grimm

LOTUS PRESS

SHANGRI-LA

Important Note:
The information and exercises introduced in this book have been carefully researched and passed on to the best of my knowledge and consciousness. Despite this fact, neither the author nor the publisher assume any type of liability for presumed or actual damages of any kind that might result from the direct or indirect application or use of the statements in this book. The information in this book is intended for interested readers and educational purposes.

First English Edition 2000
©by Lotus Press, Box 325
Twin Lakes, WI 53181, USA
The Shangri-La Series is published in cooperation
with Schneelöwe Verlagsberatung, Federal Republic of Germany
©1997 by Windpferd Verlagsgesellschaft mbH, Aitrang, Germany
All rights reserved
Translated by Christine M. Grimm
Cover design by Kuhn Graphik, Digitales Design, Zürich
Illustrations: on page 10 by Eva Wong "Feng-Shui—The Ancient Wisdom of
Harmonious Living for Modern Times" Shambala Publications Inc., Boston,
USA; on page 11 by Evelyn Lip "Chinese Geomancy—A Laymann's Guide to
Feng Shui" Times Books International, Singapore
Drawings by Heike Cobaugh, Wiesbaden/Germany
Graphics designed by Jens Mehlhase, Neumünster, executed by Uwe Hiltmann

ISBN 0914955-60-8
Library of Congress Catalog Number 00-131345

Printed in USA

Table of Contents

Preface

This book has been created from years of personal experience with feng shui. We would like to share this experience with you. Since the end of the Seventies, we have been concerned with subtle energies, which have an effect on our health. At first, we used our knowledge for ourselves, but soon we also applied it for friends and acquaintances. We eagerly collected all the information available to us and attended seminars and workshops. Our consultations gradually expanded to include all of Germany (where we live) and the neighboring countries. We held our own seminars and ultimately founded the Institute for Applied Kanyu.

This current volume shows that feng shui can have a considerably stronger influence on your health than you may have thought. During our feng shui consultations in private homes, we have repeatedly found that health problems were often the reason why people called us. The causes for health problems may very well be the influence of negative energies, as well as the lack of positive energies. The Chinese have known this for more than 3,000 years. They use two general terms for these energies in particular: "**Qi**" for positive energies and "**Sha**" for negative energies.

For our health and well-being, it is necessary that we adequately provide ourselves with positive energies. In part, we absorb these energies through our food, but we additionally take in a large part of these energies from the surrounding world through our aura. As a result, we should be sure to spend an adequate part of the day and night in an environment that contains sufficient positive energies. This is particularly important during the recuperation time at night.

Especially during sleep, it is necessary to protect ourselves from negative energies. Since we spend many hours in the same place in bed, we are exposed in a particularly concentrated way to the negative energies that may be found there. Fortunately, our body is usually capable of disintegrating the negative energies that we have absorbed during the day while we sleep. However, if we continue to absorb additional negative energies during the night, this dissolution process does not take place. To the contrary: the harmful effects of these energies are potentiated in such a manner that serious illnesses can occur.

But how can we find out whether we have created a good sleeping environment for ourselves or not? It is often possible to locate these negative energies in a very concrete way, and we will show you a method by which you can do this yourself. When we have located the various negative energies, then we can avoid them or take the appropriate protective measures. Since the possibilities of avoiding them are frequently limited, we deal extensively with protective remedies in this book.

There are some people who are capable of simply feeling these energies and invisible subtle structures. However, this generally requires a certain sensitivity coupled with a great deal of experience. If you are not one of these people, there are excellent aids for you—which we also use—called the tensor (sometimes referred to as the single-handed dowser) and the L-shaped dowsing rods (shortened to L-rods in the following text). The pendulum can also be put to good use in detecting the energies that affect us. This method is particularly successful when we want to get to know those energies or invisible structures that we want to measure as precisely as possible beforehand. We will discuss the proper use of the L-rod, tensor, and pendulum in detail in this book. It will be possible for you to understand the entire content of this book with the L-rod, tensor, or pendulum and put it to work for you in your own home.

This current volume is the **first part** of a multi-volume series on the topic of feng shui. The basic concept of this series is to extensively explore the individual fields of feng shui. In addition to the health area, feng shui can be successfully applied to promote harmonious relationships within the family, as well as in business life, among other things. At the same time, each individual volume should also provide access to the respective special topic on its own.

Introduction to Feng Shui

Feng shui comes from the Chinese and is translated to mean: "wind and water." Feng shui is the art of living in harmony with our visible and invisible surroundings. Living in harmony means health, well-being, success in our work, personal happiness, and spiritual growth.

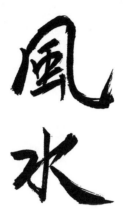

Chinese character for feng shui

In order to achieve this goal, it is necessary for us to strengthen the positive forces and avoid the negative forces. In the old advanced civilizations, including that of ancient China, people made an effort to create harmony between themselves and their surrounding world. In order to do this, it was necessary to study the laws of the visible and invisible world, applying them for the benefit of human beings. Through the specific application of the rules of feng shui, among other things, we can have a positive effect on our health and our well-being.

The art of living in harmony with our environment is based on the observation of the visible world on the one hand; on the other hand, it is also founded upon the emotional perception of the invisible world. Since not every human being has the same perceptive abilities, at an early point in time the Chinese were already concerned with giving less sensitive people reference points for judging the hidden energies of a place. From the different approaches, various "schools" of feng shui have developed. We now would like to explain these to you briefly.

The Form School

Because of their abundance of forms, the mountainous regions of southern China offered the ideal area for the development of the so-called Form School. Through observing the forms of the landscape and rivers, the ancient feng shui masters developed a very strongly differentiated evaluation of the individual forms with respect to their positive and negative impact on human beings. The interaction of the mountain forms and courses of the rivers determined the best location for a human settlement. This favorable place was also called "Xue."

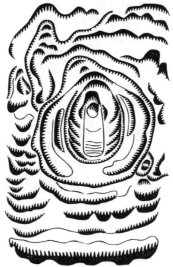

Mountain forms (old Chinese drawing)

The imperial feng shui master Yang Yun-Sang is famous for his fundamental works on the Form School, such as *The Classic on the Art of Awakening the Dragons*, *The Teaching of Approaching the Dragons*, *The Secret Meaning of the Universe*, and *The Method of the Twelve-Rung Line*. He lived from about 840-888, according to our chronology. At that time, the Form School was called *Xingshi* (shapes and forms), but today it is known by the term of *Luantou* (mountain summit).

Since the constellations of the Form School are quite diverse and their rules cannot be learned in a purely mechanical manner, the evaluation often takes place in an emotional or intuitive manner as well.

The Compass School

In general, the plains of northern China offer less criteria for the evaluation of the landscape based on forms. Already during the time of the Sung dynasty (960-1279 according to our chronology), there was an extensive system developed for evaluating a place on the basis of the influences of the directions, as well as time-related factors. Evaluating the energies of a place was done with the help of a compass (*Luopan*), which was especially developed for this purpose.

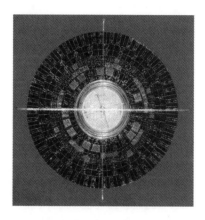

An old Chinese feng shui compass (Luopan)

Already by about 1085 according to our chronology, Shen Gua described in a book the magnetic compass and its meaning for the system of feng shui. Only after its application in feng shui evaluations was the compass also used for navigation at sea by the Chinese. The Europeans first used the compass later than the Chinese. In contrast to the European orientation of the compass needle to the north, the needle of the Chinese feng shui Luopan points south.

The Chinese feng shui scholar Wang Zhi is considered one of the main representatives of the Compass School. He lived at the time of the Sung dynasty in the north of the Fukien Province. There he wrote his main works, *Canon of the Core or the Center* and *Treatment on Questions and Answers.* An essential component of the Compass School are the astrological calculations that integrate changing influences into feng shui's way of looking at things.

The Analytical School

There are people who can directly perceive some of the influences that affect human beings at a certain place and specific time. In the process, this perception takes place through various senses. The exactness of the perception can vary greatly. It may range from a more or less indefinite feeling to a precise determination of the type and intensity of the influence. The direct perception of the energies is often also called the Intuitive School.

The path may be long, from an indefinite feeling to a concrete description of the energetic relationships at a place. In general, this requires a well-founded theoretical background in order to be able to properly classify the perceptions that have been experienced. It is good to know what energies we have actually perceived. However, it is also important to have the opportunity of repeating your own perception at a later point in time. The tensor (which is the modern form of the dowsing rod), the L-rod, or the pendulum can also be a great help to those who have a sensitive disposition in differentiating their perceptions.

A pair of L-shaped dowsing rods

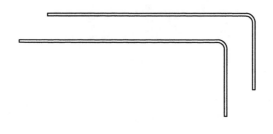

Flexible steel wire

Weight on the tip
(for example, a steel ring)

Handle

The tensor, a modern form of the dowsing rod

However, using the tensor, the L-rod, the pendulum, or another method of directly determining energies, such as kinesiology, is generally indispensable for those who have a less sensitive disposition. The classic Y-shaped dowsing rod had already been used over 4,000 years ago by the Egyptians and Chinese in order to detect things hidden from our senses. The oldest evidence of this is a law, passed by the Chinese emperor Yu from the year 2200 B.C.: Imperial officials specially trained for this purpose had to investigate plots of land intended for the construction of residential houses so that no building would be created where "evil spirits are active that bring disaster and illness with them."

We call this way of determining the qualities of a place the **Analytical School**. However, today it has been forgotten in the area of eastern and southeastern Asia. In Europe, the tensor, the pendulum, the Y-shaped dowsing rod, the L-rod, or other forms of dowsing rods, among other things, are used in detecting the strain on our health that particularly affects us in direct relation to our sleeping environment. With the tensor or pendulum, it is possible, among other things, to determine the intensity of disruptive or even positive energies. This is also important for better evaluating or modifying the results of feng shui remedies. Remedies undertaken on the basis of certain Form School situations or Compass School constellations can be done more precisely with the help of the data provided by the Analytical School.

The traditional Chinese knowledge about feng shui is not a philosophy. Instead, it is a directly comprehensible description of the relationship between the subtle energies and their effects on human beings utilizing the tensor, L-rod, pendulum, and other methods. Since the Chinese use language that is very flowery and frequently impossible for the people of the West to understand, we have made an effort to impart the ancient feng shui knowledge to you in this book in such a way that you can really apply the Analytical School in a direct manner.

Feng Shui Yesterday and Today

In order to answer certain questions, methods from all three feng shui schools are taken into account. In ancient times, the Compass School was therefore employed to clarify the question of which part of China should be the location of the capital city. The Compass School takes into account the temporally changing influences, so that the capital city has been repeatedly relocated in the history of China on the basis of these considerations. The occupation of China by the Mongolians was, among other things, attributed to not moving the capital city in time to another part of the country for reasons of convenience, even though the feng shui masters had advised this on the basis of the Compass School's criteria.

The Form School was consulted when searching for the appropriate piece of ground for building the capital city after the specific area of the country had been determined by the Compass School. Even during the age of the Shang Dynasty (1741-1122 B.C.), there is evidence that the city planning was carried out according to the feng shui criteria.

Today feng shui is routinely applied in Hong Kong, Taiwan, Singapore, Malaysia, and many other countries. For example, most architects in Hong Kong and Singapore consult a feng shui expert before beginning to construct a new building. In mainland China itself, the feng shui tradition has been preserved to this day, at least in the rural areas, despite persecution. In Japan, Kaso (as feng shui is called there) continues to be practiced up to the level of the government. The modern feng shui experts, like their predecessors in classic China, make use of all three schools mentioned here, frequently supplementing them with their own intuition and experience. Even today, most feng shui consultants in the Far East prefer to keep the precise information about their procedures to themselves. For this reason, it is often difficult for Western observers to recognize the laws of the feng shui system behind the flowery paraphrasing.

"Western" Feng Shui and Health

At no time in the past has there ever been such a complete feng shui system in the West as there has been in China. The previously existing Western knowledge has become largely lost in modern architectural development. In China, on the other hand, the effort has been made and continues to be made to translate the feng shui system to the modern way of building. The feng shui system and traditional Chinese medicine (TCM) belong together. In the West, the folk arts of healing and naturopathy have been preserved and have experienced continuous development through the past centuries. From these healing arts have come the impulses of not only looking for negative chemical or technical strains in the house but also detecting subtle energies that harm or impair the health of a human being.

Chapter 1

Detecting Energies and Subtle Structures with the Tensor, Pendulum, and L-Shaped Dowsing Rods

Work with the Tensor or Pendulum

Tensors or pendulums enable us to get a positive or negative answer to a precise question from an area of our own perception of which we are either unconscious or inadequately conscious. At the same time, this deals with making our own perceptions visible. Tensors or pendulums can therefore just show what we ourselves sense on the unconscious level. When we ask questions in the appropriate manner, we become capable of making visible our unconscious perception through a muscle reaction. We then receive a reaction from the tensor or pendulum.

Most of you will probably not have a tensor at home. However, you will probably still wish to immediately try out the practical experiments described here with a pendulum. If you do not own one, you will probably have no problem in making your own pendulum at home within five minutes. (There is a brief description of how to make your own pendulum in the appendix).

Reactions of the Tensor

Grasp the handle of the tensor with your hand. Be sure that you are not tense while doing so. If you use a tensor with a ring as a weight at the tip, the ring should be oriented in an approximately horizontal manner.

There is a limited number of possible tensor reactions (movements). So it is important to assign a clear meaning to the individual reactions of the tensor. This assignment occurs when we mentally decide what these reactions are to mean. In general, you should determine the reaction for YES and NO. But we recommend that you also determine a further reaction for NO ANSWER. In addition, we recommend assigning the up and down movement (vertical) of the pendulum to the answer YES and the movement to the left and the right (horizontal) to the answer NO. If other reactions for YES and NO, as well as NO ANSWER, have proved to be effective for you, then stick with them.

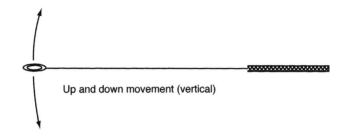

Up and down movement (vertical)

YES reaction of the tensor

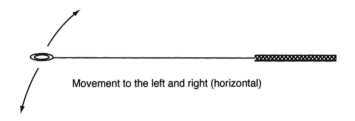

Movement to the left and right (horizontal)

NO reaction of the tensor

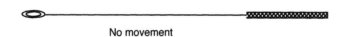

No movement

NO ANSWER reaction of the tensor

The Pendulum and Its Reaction Possibilities

You should also clearly assign YES, NO, and NO ANSWER to the pendulum swings. We recommend assigning YES to the clockwise pendulum movement and NO to the counterclockwise pendulum movement. If the pendulum remains at a standstill (no movement), we recommend that you assign NO ANSWER as its meaning. If other reactions for YES and NO, as well as NO ANSWER, have proved to be effective for you, then stick with them.

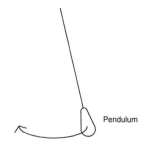

Movement in the clockwise direction

YES reaction of the pendulum

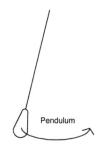

Movement in the counterclockwise direction

NO reaction of the pendulum

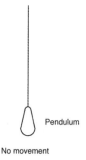

No movement

NO ANSWER reaction of the pendulum

If you do not want to do any practical experiments with the tensor or pendulum at the moment, you can continue reading Chapter 2.

Test the Tensor or Pendulum: Water or Apple Juice?

Now do a practical exercise: Take a bowl and fill it with water. Hold the tip of the tensor (the pendulum) above the water, and ask this question aloud or just in your mind: *"Is water in the bowl?"* If you have programmed yourself properly, the tensor will move up and down—vertically—and therefore show YES. (The pendulum moves clockwise). If the tensor or pendulum does not move or if it shows a different reaction, repeat the question until you receive a clear YES. If, despite repeated attempts, you only get a weak reaction or none at all, put the tensor or pendulum in the other hand and start once again. It may be that the reaction is stronger now. It is important that you basically consider a reaction to your question possible since you may otherwise block yourself.

When you have a firm grasp of this, test the NO reaction. Ask, for example: *"Is this marmalade?"* A NO reaction must now follow, which means that the tensor must move to the left and right—horizontally. (The pendulum moves in a clockwise direction.) Now ask other questions that must be answered with a no such as: "Is this apple juice?" Repeat this until you get a definite NO reaction. Then repeat this exercise with other objects until you feel sure about the NO reaction. Try to avoid asking questions with a negative response that may easily be confusing, so it is better not to ask: "Isn't this water?"!

Now determine the reaction for NO ANSWER. Ask a question like: *"What color is the water?"* Now it can only give you the response for NO ANSWER, which means that the tensor or pendulum does not move.

Measure Harmful Energies Above Swirling Water!

Those of you who have not had any previous practical experience with the tensor or pendulum should now have learned to achieve clear reactions. (YES, NO, NO ANSWER). We want to initially deal with measuring energies above flowing (swirling) water. At this point, we are interested in the energies that are harmful or disturbing for human beings.

Water Experiment I

Hold your tensor or pendulum above an opened water faucet and ask: *"Are energies above the water faucet that are harmful or disturbing for me?"* The tensor or pendulum should now indicate a YES. If you do not receive a YES, repeat these measurements several times or continue with Water Experiment II. Now turn off the faucet and ask the same question. The tensor or pendulum should now indicate a NO. Should you continue to receive a YES despite repeated measurement attempts, then you have not asked the question precisely enough in your mind. When asking about harmful or disturbing energies that have been created by *this* swirling water, we have excluded harmful or disturbing energies through swirling water of *another* origin.

The extensive formulation of questions shown here serves as practice in asking questions in precise terms. During the practical work, it is sufficient to ask the **question in a shortened form** when you are able to attune yourself to the energy that is being sought. You can, for example, ask in a shortened form: *"Are energies harmful to me because of this swirling water here?"* A person who is experienced at this will find it adequate to just become precisely attuned to the energy sought. He or she will not even have to put the question into verbal terms in the course of time. Now continue with Water Experiment II.

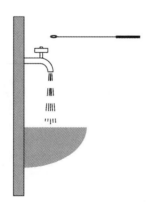

Measuring above the water faucet

Water Experiment II

Take a bowl (made of plastic, glass, or porcelain—but not of metal) and fill it with water. Then take a wooden or plastic spoon and stir it vigorously. Hold the tensor or pendulum above the moving, swirling water and ask: *"Are energies harmful to me above the bowl that have been created by this swirling water?"* The tensor or pendulum should now indicate a YES. Once the water has completely come to a standstill, repeat this question. You should now receive a NO. Should you continue to receive a YES, then you have not asked the question precisely enough in your mind. It is possible that you have measured harmful energies above a watercourse. Repeat the measurement at a different place. In addition, you can also carry out a third water experiment in a similar way with a garden hose in your yard.

Measure the Intensity of Energy Above Swirling Water!

The more intensely the water swirls, the stronger the harmful or disturbing energy will also be that emanates from it. The intensity of harmful or disruptive energy is done on a scale from 0 to 100. In this process, the value of 100 indicates the highest possible value. However, the maximum strength of the harmful or disturbing energies because of swirling water is only 30. You can find this intensity at above-ground waterfalls, for example. To determine the intensity of harmful or disruptive energies because of swirling water, you can make the following measurement:

Turn the water faucet on as far as possible and find out what intensity the harmful or disruptive energies have on the scale of 0 to 30. Hold the tensor or pendulum over the water faucet. (In the practice, it has proved helpful to already let the pendulum swing back and forth at the beginning of the measurement—which means toward you and away from you. When the YES reaction comes, the pendulum can more quickly move into a circular motion.) Ask: *"Is the intensity of the harmful energies because of this swirling water 1 or above?"* If the tensor or pendulum shows a YES, then ask: *"Is the intensity of the harmful energies because of this swirling water 2 or above?"* When you get a YES, continue increasing the number by 1 each respective time. So you ask whether the value is 1 or above, 2 or above, and so forth. When you get a NO, ask once again about the value just below it. Now you should once again get a YES. Now you have determined the intensity of the harmful or disturbing energies.

If, for example, you get the response of YES to the question of whether the intensity of the harmful energies is 20 or above, but a NO at 21 or above, then ask about 20 or above once again. Now you should once again get a YES, which means that you have determined the intensity of the harmful energies (with 20 or above, but less than 21). However, if you have once again asked about 20 or above in this example and received a NO, you have measured wrong since the intensity of the harmful energies has remained the same. Start over again.

You can also start off by steps of 5, which means from 5 or above to 10 or above and then 15 or above until you receive a NO. Then start once again with the last step and continue to count in steps of 1 as described above.

You Can Measure Subtle Structures with the L-Rod

A method for determining subtle structures that is easy to learn and dependable is finding them with the L-rod. They usually consist of an L-shaped piece of bent metal and are most often used in pairs. The long arm is generally 14 to 20 inches (35 to 50 cm) long and the short arm is 4 to 6 inches (10 to 15 cm). There are also L-rods that have the shorter arm mounted on a wooden handle or inserted into ball bearings. It is not difficult to make an L-rod. For example, you can bend copper-plated welding wire with a length of 18 to 25 inches (45 to 65 cm) to form the necessary longer and shorter arm. Welding wire with a diameter of about 1/8 inch (3 mm) is suitable. If you would like to immediately start with the experiments described here, you can also use some other form of bendable wire and make your own pair of L-rods.

The L-Rod and Its Reaction Possibilities

Hold the two short arms of the L-rod in such a way that the long arms above the hands point forward in a fairly horizontal manner.

For the reaction YES, the long arms will generally turn toward each other. For the reaction NO, the long arms will turn away from each other. For the reaction NO RESPONSE, the L-rod does not move.

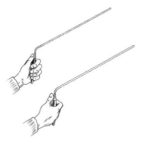

Holding the L-rod with the long arm above the hand

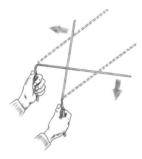

YES reaction of the L-rod (held with the long arm above the hand)

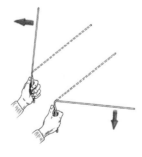

NO reaction of the L-rod (held with the long arm above the hand)

If the L-rod is held in such a way that the long arm points forward beneath the hand, the turning motion is generally reversed: it moves outward for the reaction YES and inward for the reaction NO. The reaction of NO RESPONSE remains the same.

There are also people who only work with one L-rod. If you only hold one L-rod in your right hand, with the long arm pointing forward above the hand, it will turn to the left (inward) for YES reactions and to the right (outward) for NO reactions. The L-rod does not move when there is NO RESPONSE.

Test the L-Rod in Your Home

Here is another practical exercise for you to do: Open any door in your house or apartment. Stand at least one-and-a-half yards away from this door while facing it. Hold the pair of L-rods loosely in both hands with the long arm of the each L-rod pointing forward above the hand. Now formulate your question out loud or in your mind: *"Is a subtle structure that is located in the opened door between the doorframes here?"* When you walk through the door, the answer should be YES, meaning that the two long arms of the L-rods will usually cross each other. The two long arms of the L-rods will usually cross each other either when the L-rod itself is between the doorframes or when you are there with your legs and trunk of your body. It is simply the question of whether you use the L-rod in your hands or the rest of your body for locating the subtle structure between the doorframes. A certain degree of inertia may cause the reaction of the L-rod to occur with a bit of a delay.

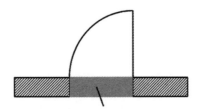

Subtle structure in the opened door between the doorframes

It is also advisable to walk through the door opening in the opposite direction in order to make a better evaluation of the delay in time (inertia of the reaction). Observe the precise spot of the reaction. When you walk through the door opening, you can optically check the position of the subtle structure in the door opening. When you search for other subtle structures, this verifiability is generally lacking. For this reason, you should repeat this measurement with other door openings so that you are very certain about your dowsing rod reactions.

If you want to look for structures with the L-rod, working with the YES reaction is usually adequate. The reaction NO RESPONSE will occur when you hold the L-rod still, meaning when it is pointing straight ahead. Use this position or reaction when you walk slowly until you find the structure you are searching for.

Search for Underground Watercourses in Your House or Garden!

Now you have learned how to find subtle structures with the L-rod. You can also find subtle structures above underground watercourses, which can be located with the L-rod.

How You Can Easily Find Underground Watercourses with the L-Rod

It is best to take a systematic approach here. First formulate the question precisely in your mind. This could be: *"Are there structures above swirling water that bring up harmful energies here?"* With this question in your head, slowly walk along the walls of the room to be measured with the L-rods. The only way to avoid overlooking a watercourse that just touches one corner of the room, for example, is by walking completely around the room once and include the door and window(s). As described above, you will generally just work with the YES response.

Look for How a Watercourse Enters and Exits with the L-Rod!

Now walk along the walls of the room or boundaries of the plot of land. If there is a watercourse running through the room (or plot of land) that you are checking, you will generally find 2 places in which your L-rod will show a YES for structures above swirling water that bring up harmful energies. Your L-rod will usually indicate a YES response as long as you are above the watercourse. The width of the watercourse can vary. When you have found a watercourse, double-check your measurement by crossing the watercourse again in the opposite direction.

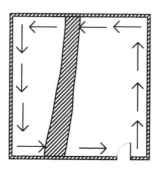

Looking for water in a room

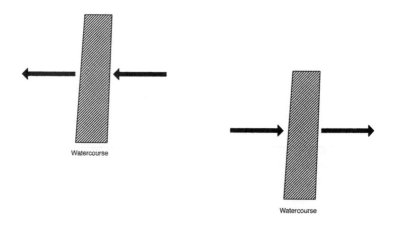

Crossing a watercourse from two sides

Determining the Path of a Watercourse
with the L-Rod

Cross the imaginary connecting line between the entrance and exit points several times. This will show you the exact course.

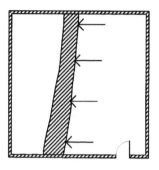

Determining the path of a watercourse in a room

You may even find more than two entrance/exit points of a watercourse. Finding three entrance/exit points of a watercourse means you have found a Y-watercourse, if you have measured correctly. This usually means that two watercourses are flowing together or a smaller one is flowing into a larger one. The crossing of watercourses is extremely rare. They occur when two watercourses at different depths (horizons) flow over each other, which implies that there is an impermeable layer between the two watercourses.

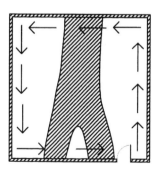

A Y-watercourse in a room

At this point, we would like to mention that there are so-called **warning stripes** on both sides of a watercourse. These warning stripes emanate at about 45 degrees from the watercourse. The distance between the watercourse and the warning stripe therefore grows with the increasing depth of the watercourse. Even if, for example, you are on the 2nd floor of a house, this distance grows about as much as the height of the first floor. In these warning stripes, you will find Trans-Sha with about 50% of the intensity of the Trans-Sha directly above the watercourse itself. The width of the warning stripe is about 8 inches (20 cm).

A Canalized Watercourse Under a Bed

On his physician's recommendation, a truckdriver had his apartment checked by a feng shui consultant. For years, he had complained about digestive problems. His physician had already been treating him with natural remedies for a longer period of time, but there had been no substantial improvements. She told him that a problem related to his sleeping area may be contributing to his digestive complaints. The feng shui consultant discovered that a canalized watercourse with a powerful swirl was located directly beneath the patient's sleeping area. It was possible to move the bed. Even after just 4 weeks, the digestive complaints had considerably improved (the naturopathic treatment had been continued as well).

How You Can Also Easily Find Underground Watercourses with the Tensor or Pendulum

While a subtle structure above a watercourse can easily be found with the L-rod, with the tensor or pendulum it is simpler to search for the so-called **carrier** of the harmful energy that is located above the watercourse. But first, here is an explanation of what we understand the carrier to be:

In order for stones to move from one place to the other, they need a carrier (or a means of transportation). Like stones, subtle energies also require a carrier to move from one place to the next.

The first step in this process is to precisely formulate the question in your mind. This could be: **"Are carriers with harmful energy above swirling water here?"** With this question in your mind, slowly walk along the walls of the room to be measured.

The Reaction of the Tensor While Walking through Rooms or Plots of Land

When searching for an underground watercourse with the tensor, the following has proved to be effective: Hold the tensor still as long as you have not found the carrier with the harmful energies for which you are searching. When you have found this carrier, the tensor will immediately show a YES. This method means that as long as you have not yet found the carrier with the harmful energies, you do not want to have a reaction from the tensor.

There is a second possibility for the tensor's reaction when you walk through the room: You put the above question into precise terms from the start. Then your tensor will show the reaction NO from the beginning, which means it will move horizontally. Here you have the reaction NO as long as you are not above a watercourse. When you have found the carrier with the harmful energies for which you are looking, the reaction will immediately change to YES.

The Pendulum Reaction While Walking through Rooms or Plots of Land

When searching for an underground watercourse with the pendulum, the following has proved to be effective: Hold the pendulum still as long as you have not yet found the carrier with the harmful energies. This means that you do not want the pendulum to react as long as you have not yet found the carrier with the harmful energies. Once you have found this carrier, the pendulum will immediately swing back and forth, which means that it moves towards you and away from you. This reaction will last until you have crossed the underground watercourse. Once you have crossed the watercourse, the pendulum will remain still once again. Should the reaction not be clear enough for you, cross the watercourse once again from the other side.

If you have a good experience with a different pendulum reaction while using the pendulum to look for an underground watercourse, then stay with this approach.

Look for How a Watercourse Enters and Exits with a Tensor or Pendulum!

Now walk along the walls of the room or the boundaries of the plot of land. If a watercourse leads through the room (or plot of land) that you are checking, you will generally find two places in which your tensor gives you a YES (or your pendulum shows a reaction) in terms of the carrier with the harmful energies because of swirling water. Your tensor will therefore generally show you a YES twice (or your pendulum will show a reaction) since the watercourse has an entrance and an exit. The width of the entrance and of the exit can vary. Once you have found a watercourse, check your measurement by crossing the watercourse in the opposite direction.

Determining the Path of a Watercourse with the Tensor or Pendulum

There are two possibilities for determining the path of a watercourse:
1) Stand with your back to the wall on the watercourse. Take the tensor or pendulum in your hand, slowly draw a semicircle with it while extending your arm in front of you and ask about carriers with harmful energies because of swirling water. This is how you can determine the width of the watercourse. Now slowly walk in the direction of the other entrance or exit point that you have determined, which will show you the path of the watercourse through the room (or plot of land) with the tensor or pendulum. If it is not possible for you to easily cover the entire width of the watercourse with a semicircular movement, then first find the right edge of the watercourse, up to the other side of the room. Determine the left edge by returning to your starting point.
2) Here is the second possibility: Cross the imaginary connecting line between the entrance and exit points several times. This will show you the exact course.

Determining the Intensity of Harmful Energies Above an Underground Watercourse with the Tensor or Pendulum

When you have found an underground watercourse, it is possible to determine the intensity of the harmful energy (in a way similar to the water experiments) with the tensor or pendulum. The maximum intensity of the harmful energies above an underground watercourse is 30. It is dependent upon the degree to which the water is swirling underground. The swirling is not equally intense above the entire watercourse and, dependent on factors like rainfall, is also subject to seasonal fluctuations.

Strain caused by swirling water is not necessarily from just one watercourse.

A Swimming Pool Beneath the Bedroom

A prosperous master craftsman bought himself a house in a distinguished neighborhood. The house had its own swimming pool, which was located directly beneath the bedroom. At first, his wife experienced muscle pain in the morning. After several weeks, she also had rheumatic joint complaints. When the master craftsman also complained about joint pain after three months, the doctor treating him advised him to call in a feng shui consultant. This consultant discovered that there was strain caused by the swimming pool located directly beneath the bedroom. In order to correct the sleeping environment, it was necessary to turn off the circulation pump of the swimming pool at night, in addition to other remedies. Even after a short time, the couple's health problems had improved.

Chapter 2

The Invisible World of Feng Shui

An Energy from Another Dimension

Perhaps you have already wondered that water is supposed to emanate harmful energies since we all know that water is both our most important food and also the elixir of life itself for the earth. So the water itself is not what emanates the harmful energies. Swirling water solely makes a process possible that brings energies from another dimension into our own dimension. But how should we understand the meaning of these other dimensions and/or our own dimension?

The term "dimension" is very complex. In general usage, dimension means something like extension, extent, or area. Perhaps you still remember the classes in art or drawing during your school days. When you draw a line, this is called the 1st dimension. The plane is called the 2nd dimension. Spatial drawing would then be the description of the 3rd dimension.

Expressed in somewhat more mathematical terms, this can be formulated as follows: We also understand the qualities of geometrical basic forms under the term "dimension." The dot is therefore dimension 0 (zero), the straight line dimension 1, the plane dimension 2, and space dimension 3. The human being cannot imagine higher dimensions in this sense. However, more than anyone before him, Einstein convinced us that there must be more than 3 dimensions.

While Einstein was still reflecting on precisely how to describe the 4th dimension, today theoretic physics even assumes that there must be more than 4 dimensions. At a renowned Parisian research institute, as a result of theoretical calculations already done ten years earlier, at the end of the 1970s scientists had already concluded that all known physical processes could only be explained if we assume that there are 7 dimensions. The teaching of feng shui also assumes that there are 7 dimensions.

The 3rd Dimension

As human beings, we live with our physical body (the body of flesh and blood) and our non-physical or subtle body (aura) in the 3rd dimension. In addition, animals and plants, the earth, our solar system, even the entire known universe exists in the 3rd dimension. Despite this, influences from other dimensions—such as astrological influences—have an effect on us. In general, these influences are characterized in that we can describe them but their mechanisms can be only examined in part at best. The Chinese already precisely registered and described these influences at a very early point in time.

The Higher Dimensions

Six further dimensions exist in addition to the 3rd. There are dimensions higher and lower dimensions than the 3rd. We call the dimensions 4, 5, 6, and 7 (in ascending order) the higher dimensions. **Time** runs increasingly more **slowly** in these higher dimensions. If, for example, we could take a trip into the 4th dimension and spend one year there, 100 years would already have passed in our 3rd dimension. Upon his return, such a "time-traveler" would no longer be greeted by his family since they would have already died by then. However, he would himself have only become one year older. So time runs slower in the 4th dimension than in the 3rd dimension. In turn, time in the 5th dimension runs more slowly than in the 4th dimension, and so forth.

The Lower Dimensions

We call the dimensions 2 and 1 (in descending order) the lower dimensions. In these lower dimensions, **time** runs increasingly **faster** than in the 3rd dimension. This means that time runs more quickly in the 2nd dimension than in the 3rd dimension. In turn, time runs even more quickly in the 1st dimension than in the 2nd dimension.

Beings that live in a higher dimension can basically imagine life in a lower dimension. So, for example, we can imagine that a being lives in a plane, such as the 2nd dimension. The other way around, it is quite difficult for a being that lives in a lower dimension to imagine life in a higher dimension. This can be illustrated through an example:

In this example, we can call the 2nd dimension Planeland. How does an inhabitant of Planeland experience our 3rd dimension. If a carrot is moved through Planeland, its inhabitants will see an orange-colored circle appearing out of the blue and becoming increasingly larger. The orange circle finally turns into a green circle, which then disappears once again.

We would have a similar experience if we were in the 4th dimension. We would only recognize three-dimensional "cross-sections" of the four-dimensional world.

The rest of the qualities that a higher or a lower dimension has are usually difficult to explain. Through our perception and our wealth of experience, we are only familiar with experiences from the 3rd dimension. However, we are still exposed to influences from other dimensions. In this process, the influences from the 4th and 5th dimensions are most important for the system of feng shui.

Energies Change Between the Dimensions

Neither the positive nor the negative energies of feng shui constantly exist in the 3rd dimension, even though this may initially appear to be the case to us. Instead, they change their dimensions at the so-called **points of intersection**. The energies important for our health and well-being change from the 4th or 5th dimension into our 3rd dimension. However, these energies are only making a "guest appearance" here, although they are tremendously important for us during this period of time. We will give you more extensive information about their effect upon us during the course of this book.

They end their guest appearance in our 3rd dimension by once again disappearing into a higher dimension (4th or 5th dimension). Although their manner of changing back and forth between the dimensions eludes our perception, we can still precisely describe and locate these points of intersection.

The "Invisible" World Has 32 Levels

The Visible and the "Invisible" World

The influences of feng shui energies from higher dimensions have greatly differentiated effects on human beings and their environment. In order to intensify positive energies or reduce—or even eliminate—negative energies, we need a more precise knowledge of the laws regarding how these energies can have a concrete effect on us. So we must now therefore deal with a bit of theory.

In our 3rd dimension there are not only the things that we can see, hear, taste, smell, or touch. As a result, in the 3rd dimension our body exists of more than flesh and blood. In addition to this visible, material body there is also our non-material body in the form of the aura; however, this is not visible for most people. Yet, the visible and non-visible body belong together and form one unity. This not only applies to the body of human beings, but also to animals and plants, which also have an aura. This even applies to rocks and all of matter in our 3rd dimension. In addition, there are many invisible "things" that only exist in the invisible range. Since most people can only directly perceive what is visible, they sometimes tend to consider the invisible as being non-existent. Then it is even more difficult to perceive the invisible world in a differentiated way.

Is a Window Glass Red, Blue, and Green at the Same Time?

Three clairvoyants receive the assignment of describing what invisible things there are for them "to see" in a room. The first clairvoyant sees the pane of glass as red, the second sees it as blue, and the third sees it as green. So who is right?

Our tip for readers who are clairvoyant: Look to see what color the window glass is. It is possible that you see the window glass in none of the three colors mentioned, but rather in a milky white? How can this be explained? You are probably right, in addition to the three clairvoyants, but you have all programmed yourselves in a different way. Either you have perceived different energies that actually each have a different respective color. Or it may also be that you or other clairvoyants have actually seen the color of the glass on different invisible levels*. These planes can also be called degrees of fineness.

In contrast to the visible area, a pane of glass, for example can exist simultaneously on various levels in the non-visible area. In concrete terms: In the visible area, the same pane of glass is simultaneously clearly transparent (without color), but in the non-visible area it is also red, green, blue, and milky-white. We could say that in

---

* Levels should not be understood as different heights in space here.

addition to the visible world, there are several different non-visible "worlds" that exist at the same time.

The Human Being is Invisible on 32 Levels

In the invisible range, we count a total of 32 levels. However, for our topic it is not necessary to discuss the special qualities of each individual level. In individual cases, it is helpful for our health to become more familiar with some of the levels. Our non-visible body, our aura, exists on these 32 different levels as well. The energies that are important for our health also have an effect on us on a total of 32 levels.

You Have Already Measured on the 2nd Level

Without knowing it, when you attempted to measure the intensity of the energy above the swirling water, you measured on the 2nd level. For swirling water, the energy is usually the most intense on the 2nd level; in addition, the energy of the 2nd level has the strongest effect on the human being here.

We give the numbers 1 to 32 to the 32 levels for the sake of simplicity. The numbering has not been chosen randomly; instead, it orients itself toward the degree of fineness in relation to the other levels.

If we would consider what is visible to be the visible level, it would be the coarsest of all levels. But we do not want to include it in the following list of the levels. The 32 invisible levels are finer than the visible level; however, they can also be organized according to their different degrees of fineness.

The first invisible level is the coarsest. The second level is finer than the first. When we say "fine," we could also use the term "more subtle" here. We can therefore say that the second level is **subtler** than the first. Up to and including the level 10, the individual levels become increasingly subtle. Starting at level 11, the degree of fineness has increased to the point that we do no longer want to call the 11th level "subtle" but say that it is "**non-material**." The 11th level is therefore less material than the 10th level. The degrees of fineness also continue to increase after the 11th level so that the 12th level is once again less material or finer than the 11th level.

The Chinese Call Structures "Li"

The term "Li" is employed in a more extensive sense than the word "structure" in English. For example, geography is called "Di Li" (translated as: the structures of the earth) in Chinese. This term also includes the energetic pathways within the body (for example, acupuncture meridians) and the finest thought structures. From acupuncture we know that the structures described there are not only meant to explain the interrelations as a philosophical concept, but are used in a very real sense; for example, by applying needles, moxa therapy, acupressure, among other things, to achieve concrete results. When we use the term Li in the system of feng shui, we mean the invisible structures upon which the energies and their carriers move.

The interplay of structures (Li), carriers, and energy can be explained by the following example:

When there is a river, boats, tree trunks, or other objects can swim or float on it. The boats, tree trunks, and other swimming objects would be the visible energy that is transported by the river (the carrier). The river itself moves within the riverbed (the structure Li).

Direction-Dependent Structures

Carriers and energies use subtle and non-material direction-dependent structures, among other things. These structures generally have clearly definable geometric forms such as the cube.

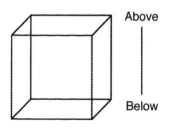

Individual cube

These structures are normally hidden from the human eye. However, the cubes can be easily found by means of the L-rod, tensor, or pendulum. Looking for them is not considerably different from searching for underground watercourses.

Cube Systems

The most important direction-dependent structures have the form of adjoining rows of cubes and are therefore also called cube systems. As a result, the individual cubes are arranged in rows directly next to each other, as well as above and below each other. These cube systems can be found throughout the entire earth, reaching both above the earth into the heights and into the earth itself. We find them in the open countryside, as well as within houses. The cube systems are often named after the average side length or height of the individual cube. In the open countryside, the side walls are oriented toward the **north-south and east-west** or diagonally and are directed vertically upward at the same time. The direction is based on the feng shui direction of north, which deviates 2.6 degrees to the west from the geographic direction of north (the 3rd dimension). The feng shui direction of north itself or the feng shui North Pole is a direction in the 4th dimension, which is constant for all latitudes. There has been no extra note made of it in the graphics with the cube systems since the "N" is related to the feng shui direction of north. The thickness of the side walls of the cube is different in the individual cube systems.

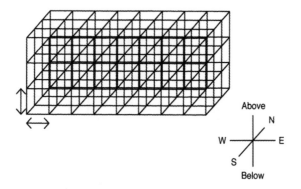

A cube system consists of individual cubes with approximately the same size. The upper and lower boundary of the cubes is on a horizontal level. The cube systems are frequently named according to the average length of the side or height of the individual cube (see arrow).

The 0.67-Centimeter System

The 0.67-Centimeter System is the fundamental cube system upon which the other, larger cube systems are oriented in principle. In the open countryside, it is oriented in a north-south and east-west direction. The average length of the side and the height of the cube consist of approx. 2/8 inches (exactly 0.67 cm). Special geological formations (such as faults and ore storage sites) can lead to a deviation from the north-south or east-west course of the side walls.

The 0.95-Centimeter Systems A and B

The 0.95-Centimeter System A runs diagonally in the 0.67 Centimeter System. The side lengths consist of approx. 3/8 inches (exactly 0.95 cm) and the height is approx. 2/8 inches (exactly 0.67 cm) so that the horizontal surfaces are identical with the horizontal surfaces of the 0.67-Centimeter System.

The 0.95-Centimeter System B also runs diagonally in the 0.67 Centimeter System. The side lengths are also approx. 3/8 inches (exactly 0.95 cm) here. However, the height is also approx. 3/8 inches (exactly 0.95 cm) so that the horizontal surfaces are not identical with the horizontal surfaces of the 0.67-Centimeter System.

The larger diagonal cube systems are oriented upon the 0.95 Centimeter System A and B in principle

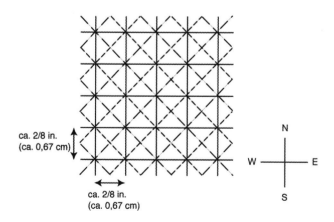

The 0.95-Centimeter Diagonal Systems A and B (each with different broken lines) and the 0.67-Centimeter System (solid lines).

Direction-Dependent Structures in the House

In parallelepiped-shaped houses that have their own aura structure (starting at a minimum volume of about 180 cubic meters or 235 cubic yards), the orientation of the 0.67-Centimeter System adapts approximately to the alignment of the room walls or the house diagonals. This means that the larger cube systems will also align themselves accordingly, whereby additional deviations because of metals and electromagnetic influences may occur.

Direction-Dependent Structures in a House that Deviates Less than 22.5 Degrees from the Feng Shui Direction of North

In houses that deviate from 0 to 22.5 degrees from the feng shui direction of north, the orientation of the 0.67-Centimeter System adapts approximately to the direction of the house.

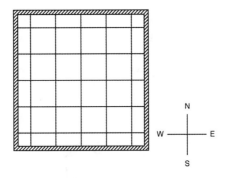

Symbolic depiction showing the course of the 0.67-Centimeter System in a house with its walls oriented toward the feng shui direction of north. For a house with dimensions of 33 x 33 feet (10 x 10 m), this would mean, for example, that only every three-hundredth line is depicted.

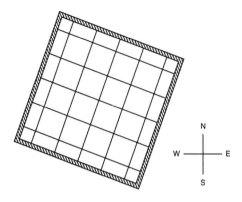

The 0.67-Centimeter System in a house with its walls that deviates less than 22.5 degrees from the feng shui direction of north. In this example, the house is turned 20 degrees clockwise in comparison to the feng shui direction of north.

Direction-Dependent Structure in a House that Deviates 22.5 to 45 Degrees from the Feng Shui Direction of North

In houses that deviate 22.5 to 45 degrees from the feng shui direction of north, the orientation of the 0.67-Centimeter System adapts itself approximately to the alignment of the house diagonals.

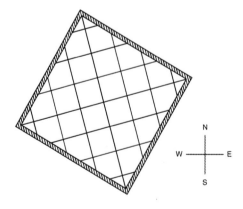

The 0.67-Centimeter System in a house with a square floor plan, which deviates 22.5 to 45 degrees from the feng shui direction of north with its walls. In this example, the house is turned 30 degrees clockwise in comparison to the feng shui direction of north.

In houses that do not have a square floor plan, a shearing of the side walls occurs so that they no longer meet at right angles.

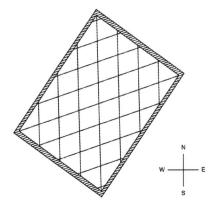

The 0.67-Centimeter System in a house with a square floor plan, which deviates from 22.5 to 45 degrees from the feng shui direction of north with its wall. A shearing of the 0.67-Centimeter System occurs. In this example, the house is turned 30 degrees clockwise in comparison to the feng shui direction of north.

Formation of House Diagonals in L-Shaped or Elongated Houses

In L-shaped houses, the house diagonals are shaped as if the floor plan would be extended to form an imaginary rectangle. The imaginary rectangle usually includes a directly adjoining garage, but not a carport.

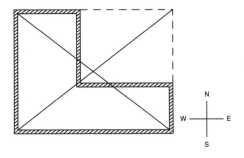

Formation of house diagonals in an L-shaped house

In elongated houses with a rectangular floor plan, the length of whose sides deviate no more than 1:2.2 from each other, the house diagonal is formed for the entire floor plan. The 0.67-Centimeter System therefore shears up to a maximum of 50 to 130 degrees. When the ratio of the side length exceeds 1:2.2, the rectangular floor plan is divided into two rectangles of approximately equal size (max. difference of 3:4) with their own diagonals. When the two large rectangles tend to be unequal, the course of the 0.67-Centimeter System is parallel to the average value of the two angles of the somewhat differing diagonals.

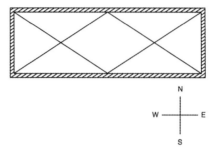

Formation of the house diagonals in an elongated house. In this case, the house diagonals form through two equally large rectangles.

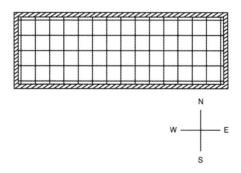

In this case, the 0.67-Centimeter System runs parallel to the house walls.

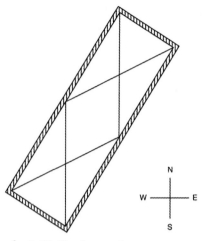

In this case, the 0.67-Centimeter System runs parallel to the house diagonals. In this example, the house is turned 30 degrees clockwise in comparison to the feng shui direction of north.

Houses with side lengths that deviate more than 1:4.9 from each other form 3—instead of 2—individual squares, which are also approximately equal in size. On the other hand, the course of the 0.67-Centimeter System in somewhat unequal large rectangles is parallel to the average value of the angle of the somewhat differing diagonals.

Negative Energies in Cube Walls Harm Our Health

The cube systems are particularly significant for our health. Energies that are negative for human beings are conducted into the side walls of certain larger cube systems. These negative energies are also called "Sha." We can easily imagine that we frequently walk through the side walls of these cube systems or spend shorter or longer periods of time "within" them during the day. Fortunately, a human being can tolerate quite a lot of the Sha that is found within these side walls, in as far as he or she has the opportunity of dissolving it in an unencumbered sleeping area during the night. Only when a person is also exposed to this Sha during the night because he or she sleeps within such cube walls can disruptions of well-being or even serious health disorders arise. We will introduce these cube systems, which are important for our health, and the illnesses related to them in this volume.

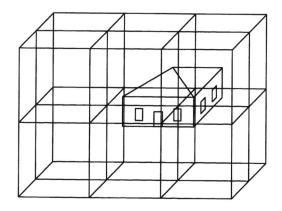

A house in the cube system: We also find the cube walls inside a house.

Chapter 3

Trans-Sha, Geo-Sha, and Per-Sha

Trans-Sha that Comes from Below

How Is the Hartmann (Cube) System Related to Watercourses?

Mr. M had just learned how to look for water with the tensor. Since he was thinking of buying a house, he paid attention to underground watercourses when he looked at them. Even at the first house he looked at, he noticed that he could find a watercourse every two meters. He decided not to buy the house. When the same thing happened to him as he looked at the next house, he began to doubt the results. A friend of his, who is a healing practitioner, explained to him: "You didn't find a watercourse but the side walls of the Hartmann System."

The Hartmann System

The Hartmann System is an abbreviation for the Hartmann Cube System. It was first described by the German physician Dr. E. Hartmann. If we only look at the flat surface of the Hartmann System (meaning the places where it goes through the earth's surface or the ceiling of the room), a grid structure appears. This is why the Hartmann System is also frequently called the Hartmann Grid. The distance of the side walls of the Hartmann System consists of approx. 6 1/2 feet (6 to 7 1/2 ft.) or 2 meters (1.8 to 2.3 m) in the north-south direction and approx. 8 1/2 feet (6 1/4 to 9 ft.) or 2.50 meters (1.9 to 2.7 m) in the east-west direction. The height of the individual cube consists of approx. 6 1/2 feet (2 m). The side walls of the Hartmann System have an average width of 2 to 7 inches (6 to 18 cm).

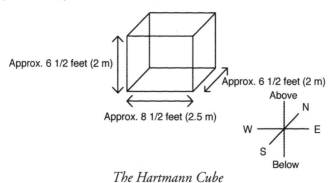

The Hartmann Cube

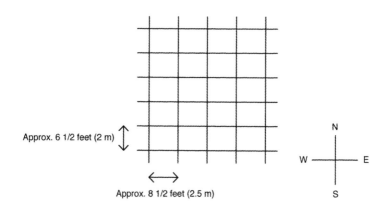

The Hartmann System (top view)
Since the Hartmann System looks like a grid when seen from above, it is also called the Hartmann Grid.

Mr. M. had not been all that wrong. The same energy rises in the side walls of the Hartmann System as does above watercourses. However, the precondition for this is that an underground watercourse passes through the side walls of the nearby Hartmann System.

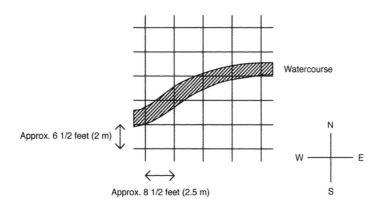

A watercourse in the Hartmann System (top view): the intensity of the energies in the side walls of the Hartmann System is dependent upon the closest watercourse and decreases with increasing distance from the watercourse.

How Is the Energy Created Above an Underground Watercourse?

The energy above an underground watercourse is an energy of the 5th dimension that has reached our dimension through swirling water. This energy moves more slowly in the 5th dimension than in our dimension, the 3rd. When it reaches our dimension, it becomes faster. We therefore call this process **acceleration**. If we could perceive the direction of flow for this energy of the 5th dimension in our dimension, we would say this is an energy that comes from the side. We call it **Trans-Sha**.

What is Trans-Sha?
Trans-Sha is an energy that is harmful to human beings. We find it above underground watercourses (swirling water), as well as in the side walls of the Hartmann and the 170-Meter System. Trans-Sha can also be activated through metals (see *Trans-Sha Also Comes from the Side* on page 56 ff.

The swirling water of an underground watercourse activates invisible subtle intersection points for Trans-Sha. the intersection points are necessary so that Trans-Sha can be accelerated from the 5th dimension into the 3rd dimension. They have the form of a spiral with a hole in the center. The spirals are located vertically in the side walls of the Hartmann System: however, they can also be found above swirling water. They not only bring Trans-Sha into our dimension, but also effect **an upward change in the direction of flow.**

Trans-Sha rises vertically both above a watercourse, as well as in the side walls of the Hartmann System. So when we stand on the ground or floor of a room, the Trans-Sha comes out of the ground or from below. For this reason, the Trans-Sha energy is occasionally also called earth emanations or earth rays.

A Couple Sleeps in the Side Wall of a Hartmann System for 20 Years

This is what an experienced feng shui consultant discovered: "I still have a very good recollection of the first time I checked a sleeping environment: A retired couple had lived in a housing-development home close to the city of Kassel, Germany for 20 years. They told me that two years after they moved in, the wife first experienced kidney pains. After med-

ical treatment, the pain initially went away. Instead, pain occurred in her back. During the following period of time, the kidney and back pains alternated repeatedly without medical treatment bringing any lasting success. When examining the sleeping area, I discovered that the couple slept in a side wall of the Hartmann System that ran directly through the kidney area and the painful parts of her back. Just a few days after correcting the sleeping area, there was considerable improvement of the complaints. A typical characteristic for the harmful effect of Trans-Sha in the side walls of the Hartmann System is that it takes about two years for the first complaints to occur."

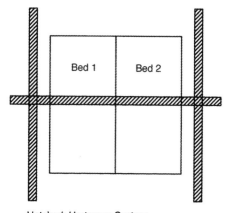

Hatched: Hartmann System

A double bed in a side wall of the Hartmann System

Determining the Side Walls of the Hartmann System with the L-Rod

The simplest way of finding the subtle structure of the side walls of the Hartmann System is with an L-rod. If you want to estimate the direction in which the Hartmann System runs in a room, it is advisable to first determine the orientation of the house in relation to the geographic direction of north or the feng shui direction of north (see section on *Direction-Dependent Structures* on page 39 ff). Then you can foresee whether the side walls of the Hartmann System run parallel to the house walls or the house diagonals.

If, in houses (with parallel house walls), you can evaluate that the side walls of the Hartmann System run parallel to the house walls, it is best to walk parallel to the house walls when searching for the side walls. Then you will cross the side walls of the Hartmann System. If you can evaluate that the side walls of the Hartmann System run parallel to the house diagonals, it is best to walk at an right angel to the house diagonals when searching for the side walls. Then you will also cross the side walls of the Hartmann System. Walk through the area with the following question: *"Is a side wall of the Hartmann System here?"* You can also search for the side walls of the Hartmann System with the tensor or pendulum using this question. If Trans-Sha is conducted from below to above in the side walls of the Hartmann System in a noticeable intensity, it is usually simpler to use a different question.

Measuring the Carrier of Trans-Sha in the Side Walls of the Hartmann System with the Tensor or Pendulum

When we look for Trans-Sha in the side walls of the Hartmann System, we can asked about **Trans-Sha**, the **carrier**, or the **direction-dependent structure** by using a tensor or pendulum. It has also proved effective in the practice to ask about the carrier. The formulation of the question here is: *"Are carriers that conduct Trans-Sha into the side walls of the Hartmann System here?"* This way of asking the question may appear to be complicated and time-consuming. However, it creates precise programming in your search for Trans-Sha. When you are sure that you have programmed yourself precisely, you can simplify the question and just ask: *"Is Trans-Sha in the side walls of the Hartmann System here?"* Since the carrier of Trans-Sha in the side walls of the Hartmann System is the same as the carrier of Trans-Sha above a watercourse, it will be easy for you to find the side walls of the Hartmann System.

Determining the Intensity of Trans-Sha in the Side Walls of the Hartmann System

When you have found the side walls of the Hartmann System, it is possible to determine the intensity of the Trans-Sha in the side walls with a tensor or pendulum. You are already familiar with the determination of intensity from the water experiments and/or from the section on underground watercourses. The intensity of the energies in the side walls of the Hartmann System is dependent upon the closest watercourse. It diminishes with increasing distance from the watercourse. The maximum intensity of Trans-Sha in the side walls of the Hartmann System is 30.

Trans-Sha Is Also in the Walls of the 170-Meter System

We find Trans-Sha not only above swirling water and in the side wall of the Hartmann System, but also in the side walls of an additional direction-dependent cube system, the 170-Meter cube System, abbreviated into the 170-Meter System. This system was first described by Wilhelm Gerstung. Its side walls have a thickness of 4–8 inches (10–20 cm). Similar to the Hartmann System, there are also spirals located in the side walls at intersection points that accelerate Trans-Sha of the 5th dimension into the 3rd dimension. The conduction of Trans-Sha also takes place vertically with an upward direction in the side walls of the 170-Meter System. It is important to know that, in contrast to the Hartmann System, the existence of Trans-Sha in the 170-Meter System is not dependent upon the existence of an underground watercourse.

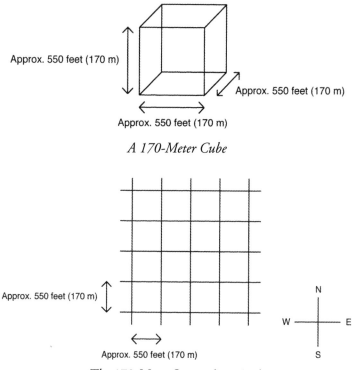

Approx. 550 feet (170 m)

Approx. 550 feet (170 m)

Approx. 550 feet (170 m)

A 170-Meter Cube

Approx. 550 feet (170 m)

Approx. 550 feet (170 m)

N

W ——|—— E

S

The 170-Meter System (top view).
The distance between the side walls is approx. 550 feet
(500 to 625 ft.) or 170 meters (150 to 190 m).

For the sake of simplicity, we have called it the 170-Meter System up to now. However, there are two 170-Meter Systems that have the same characteristics. You will therefore also find both systems equally by asking the questions. This means that you will find an additional side wall of a different 170-Meter System between the two side walls of the first 170-Meter System. This additional side wall will be located at about the halfway point.

Measuring Trans-Sha in the Side Walls of the 170-Meter System with the L-Rod, Tensor, or Pendulum

For the **170-Meter System**, proceed in a way similar to that described under the sections on underground watercourses or the Hartmann System. When searching with the L-rod, the question to ask is: *"Is the side wall of a 170-Meter System with Trans-Sha here?"* When using the tensor or pendulum, the question is: *"Are carriers that conduct Trans-Sha into the side walls of a 170-Meter System here?"* The maximum intensity of Trans-Sha in the 170-Meter System is once again 30. If you are simply searching for the side wall of a 170-Meter System without tuning in to a side wall with Trans-Sha, you may find the side walls of two additional 170-Meter Systems that do not conduct Trans-Sha and are therefore without significance here.

Trans-Sha Also Comes from the Side

Up to now, we have become familiar with the Trans-Sha found above water and conducted upward into the side walls of the Hartmann and 170-Meter System. Unfortunately, through our modern way of building and furnishing we create an abundance of situations that bring this Trans-Sha, which is harmful to us, from the side into our living rooms and bedrooms. How is this possible?

Metals Determine the Direction

Since the Industrial Revolution, it has been customary primarily in the West to use many metals for both construction purposes and interior furnishing. Metals in the side walls of the Hartmann or the 170-Meter System change the way that the spirals function in their side walls. The spirals initially accelerate Trans-Sha of the 5th dimension into our dimension, as described above. However, there is no upward change of the direction of flow. Instead, Trans-Sha largely maintains its horizontal direction of flow.

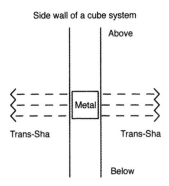

Metal brings Trans-Sha into our dimension

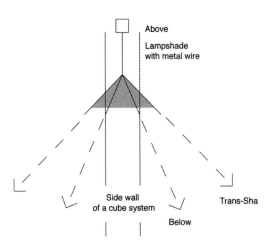

Dependent upon the form of the metal, in the 3rd dimension Trans-Sha can also be directed toward where the tip or projecting parts of a metal object point.

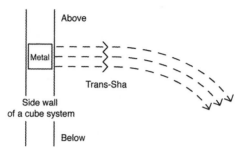

An arc-shaped path may be found when there is a longer distance.

When the Trans-Sha of the 3rd dimension meets further metal objects, these metals activate additional spirals of the Hartmann System so that Trans-Sha is once again accelerated from a higher dimension into the 3rd dimension. This process is also called the *Ping-Pong effect.*

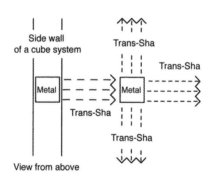

Ping-pong effect

Trans-Sha Can Also Penetrate Room Walls

Penetration is dependent upon the wall's thickness and the construction materials employed. The size and form of the metal also play a role. Trans-Sha that has been activated by large and heavy metal objects frequently is capable of penetrating a room wall, but the penetration of two room walls occurs less often. On the other hand, Trans-Sha that has been activated by small and light metal objects rarely penetrates normal room walls. A light wall construction provides less protection than solid masonry. Walls made of reinforced concrete with rebar are also less likely to be penetrated. However, be sure there are no nails in the wall.

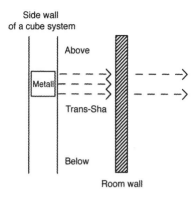

Trans-Sha can also penetrate room walls.

Metals in the Side Walls of the 10-Meter and 250-Meter System

Further important cube systems are the 10-Meter and the 250-Meter Cube System, also abbreviated to the 10-Meter and 250-Meter System. (These cube systems are discussed in detail in the section *Sick Because of Geo-Sha?*, on page 64 ff.) They normally have nothing to do with Trans-Sha. However, if metals are put into their side walls, the Trans-Sha that then occurs is usually twice as strong as that of the Hartmann or 170-Meter System. This can very well lead to substantial health disorders. The German naturopath Andreas Kopschina was the first to describe the problems that result when metals are placed in the side walls of the 10-Meter System. Typical interior furnishing objects made of metal described in the following section, as well as the permanently installed metal objects described further below, can activate Trans-Sha in the walls of the 170-Meter and the Hartmann System, as well as in the walls of the 10-Meter and 250-Meter System.

A 15-Year-Old Girl No Longer Wets Her Bed

A feng shui consultant had the following story to tell: "A healing practitioner called me and asked whether bed-wetting could be caused or intensified by a feng shui problem. An older woman from her village, who was receiving treatment from her, had asked what could be done about the bed-wetting of her 15-year-old granddaughter. The doctors had not been able to help up to now and her daughter-in-law was horribly ashamed of the situation.

When I ultimately carried out the examination of the home, only the grandmother was present. She told me that her daughter-in-law knew nothing of the appointment and had even tried to expressly prohibit her from having a feng shui consultant come. The bed itself did not stand at a cube side wall, but a mirror was located in a side wall of the 10-Meter System and the entire surface of the mirror extensively emanated toward the bed. Together with the grandmother, I moved the mirror in such a way that it no longer stood in the side wall of the 10-Meter System, but also so that nothing seemed suspicious to the mother. About four weeks later, the healing practitioner called me to say that the bed-wetting had stopped."

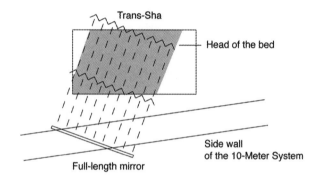

A full-length mirror in a side wall of the 10-Meter System.

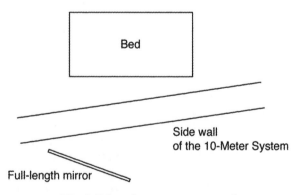

The full-length mirror was moved.

Too Many Metals in the Bedroom

If there is a side wall of the 10-Meter System in your bedroom, the entire bedroom is frequently negatively affected by Trans-Sha because of metals that are used today.

There are particular **furnishing and decoration objects** that can cause problems in your bedroom. They are mirrors (closets with mirrors on the doors), metal beds (when the metal projects beyond the frame), ceiling lamps, lighting strips, ceiling reflecting lamps, halogen lighting equipment on wires or metal tracks, nightstand lamps of metal (such as a metal base or lampshade with wire latticework), floor lamps, light fittings of bedroom closets, clock radios, telephones or cell phones next to the bed, television sets, video recorders, stereos, metal clothes trees and stands (including those on wheels), metal chairs and shelves, all-metal closets, metal designer furniture, and refrigerators.

The following objects can also cause problem: metal picture frames, copper pictures, cashboxes, large jewelry cases (such as those in nightstands), decorative objects made of metal (such as metal figurines), metal (decorative) plates, pewter pitchers, copper pitchers, watering cans of copper or brass, flower vases of metal (such as copper), flower pots of metal (such as brass), tin cans, trash cans, and wastepaper baskets of metal.

Keys in closet doors, drawers, and room doors can, when they are located in the side walls of the 10-Meter or 250-Meter System, have an extremely strong effect since they may line up precisely with the sleeping person. This effect is particularly strong when the affected person has the habit of not changing sleeping positions.

Clothes rails of metal, particularly in combination with wire hangers or all-metal clothes hangers can, when the hangers point toward the sleeping person, trigger a negative impact because of Trans-Sha.

The bedroom in our age has also frequently become a **storeroom** for a great variety of metal objects: ironing boards, irons, metal laundry racks, sewing machines, home trainers, and other training equipment made of metal (such as weights), typewriters and other office machines, vacuum cleaners, ladders, tools, tripods, cameras and film projectors, sets of cooking pots, backpacks with steel frames, old office machines and computers, old radios and televisions, etc. In our examinations, we also found ping-pong tables with metal frames, bicycles, coin collections, silverware, microwave ovens, toasters, weapons, old washing machines, etc.

A great many metal toys can be found in **children's rooms**. Among these are tricycles, children's bicycles and scooters, pedal cars, doll carriages, electric trains, and remote-controlled cars. Baby carriages, strollers, and buggies are also frequently placed in children's rooms by the parents. Playpens with metal frames are also among the objects that activate Trans-Sha.

Metal Beds

Metal beds activate Trans-Sha for the sleeping person particularly when the metal head or foot parts of the bed are higher than the bed frame. In this case, Trans-Sha with a great intensity is created when, for example, the head or foot end of the bed is located in a side wall of the 10-Meter System. Among the metal beds are also the so-called hospital beds brought into the home especially for sick persons or other patients requiring care. Beds with electrical motors, in addition to a possible negative impact through electrosmog, can also lead to problems with Trans-Sha. Fortunately, **inner-spring mattresses** and bed frames of metal are rarely a source of Trans-Sha for the sleeping person since it tends to runs downward at the side or diagonally in these cases. **Electric blankets** should be viewed similarly to inner-spring mattresses in relation to Trans-Sha. However, the strain because of electrosmog should also be taken into consideration.

Permanently Installed or Mounted Metal Objects

Metal objects such as metal and metal-reinforced synthetic windows, metal window-sills, door and window handles of metal, metal blinds, metal jalousies, curtain rods of metal, safes, ceiling ventilators, tanning beds, thermostats of heaters, as well as other metal parts that project out of the wall (including nails!) frequently bring Trans-Sha into the room and therefore to the sleeping area or other places in which we spend a greater amount of time. Eaves, gutters of metal, balcony railings, cellar gratings, and other metal parts of larger dimensions attached to the outside of the house, such as **satellite dishes** and roof antennas, as well as exterior paneling of aluminum or another metal, can also bring Trans-Sha into the interior of the house.

Aluminum or Plastic Blinds?

A feng shui consultant points out the special characteristics of a sleeping environment at night: "A businessman, 45 years old, had suffered a sudden loss of hearing. His family doctor told him that the cause was certain to be stress, so that not much improvement could be expected in his case. A naturopathic doctor, whom he consulted afterward, advised him to call a feng shui consultant since feng shui problems often play a role in the sudden loss of hearing or tinnitus (ringing in the ears). My examination initially had a negative result. However, as I said goodbye, his wife was just letting down the aluminum shade. We went back into the bedroom. Now an illness-causing Trans-Sha could clearly be measured in the room with the tensor. Despite a continuing fear of possible burglary, from that point on they did not lower the aluminum blinds. His complaints improved at an astonishing rate. Later, the aluminum blinds were replaced by plastic blinds since the couple continued to fear a burglary."

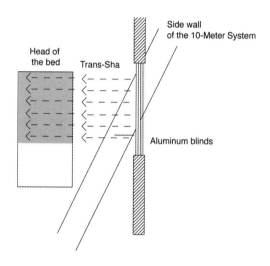

Aluminum blinds activate Trans-Sha.

Underfloor Heating

Because of the swirling water, underfloor heating with warm water leads to a negative impact because of Trans-Sha in the entire room and in the rooms above. The average intensity of the negative impact is about 8 (on the familiar scale of 0 to 100). Plastic pipes, copper pipes, and high-grade steel pipes are used for this purpose. For copper pipes and high-grade steel pipes, no additional problems with Trans-Sha worth mentioning occur because of metal. However, in the section on *Vital-Qi* on page 107 we will discuss other problems of underfloor heating in relation to copper and high-grade steel pipes.

Lenses Have a Stronger Effect than Spirals

The two case examples with serious disorders because of badly placed metal are typical for the side walls of the 10-Meter System. In the side walls of the 10-Meter System, as well as the 250-Meter System, we do not find spirals but lenses that accelerate Trans-Sha from the 5th dimension because of metal.

Sick Because of Geo-Sha?

What is Geo-Sha?
Geo-Sha is an energy harmful to human beings, found in the side walls of certain direction-dependent cube systems all over the world.

Have you already had personal experience with Geo-Sha? Did you sleep well the past few nights? Did you wake up at night even though you set no alarm? Do you feel tired and exhausted in the morning, even if you slept eight hours? Do you sleep better when on vacation or staying at a friend's place than you do at home? If you have problems with your nightly sleep or chronic health disorders, you may, without knowing it, already have had personal experience with Geo-Sha.

What is Geo-Sha?

Geo-Sha is an energy that has a similar effect on human beings as Trans-Sha, with which you are now familiar. We find Geo-Sha in the side walls of certain direction-dependent cube systems. The **10-Meter System** and the **250-Meter System** are particularly important for our health. Like Trans-Sha, Geo-Sha is also an energy from a higher dimension that has reached our dimension. In this case, this has occurred through a lens. However, in contrast to Trans-Sha, this energy has a different direction of flow in the 5th dimension. It also behaves differently in our dimension than Trans-Sha.

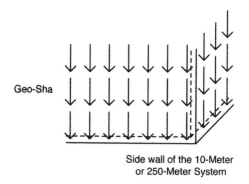

Geo-Sha

Side wall of the 10-Meter
or 250-Meter System

*Course of Geo-Sha in the side walls of the 10-Meter and
250-Meter System.*

The 10-Meter System

The 10-Meter System (also named the Benker Cube System or Benker System after its discoverer Anton Benker of Starnberg/Germany) is a direction-dependent structure that occurs everywhere on earth. Because its average side length and height of the cube is 10 meters (approx. 3.3 feet), it is called the 10-Meter System. The average length of a side can fluctuate between approx. 27 feet (8 m) and 36 feet (11 m). The side walls of the cube have a thickness of 4 to 24 inches (10 to 60 cm). The Geo-Sha, which is harmful to human beings, is conducted from above to below in its side walls. It has been frequently observed that larger metal objects in the interior decoration, as well as in the construction, of a house can lead to a spreading of the side walls of the 10-Meter System. The individual 10-meter side walls may then appear as doubled or even tripled side walls. Then the individual walls will run relatively close to each other.

Metal objects can also lead to a displacement of the normal course of the 10-Meter System. This is particularly significant in the case of moveable metal objects. For example, a car parked next to the house overnight can shift the side wall of a 10-Meter System into the bed during the night; this would not be evident when the situation is examined during the day. A sewing machine that is placed in a different location during the night than during the day may also have a similar effect. In its course, the Hartmann System adapts in part to the path of the 10-Meter System. In the side walls of the 10-Meter System, or directly next to them, one side wall of the Hartmann System can be found.

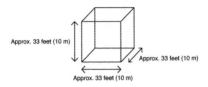

The 10-Meter Cube

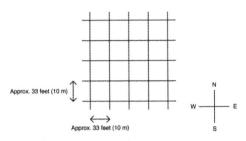

The 10-Meter System (top view)

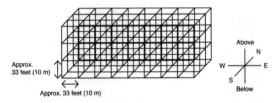

The 10-Meter System

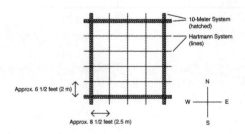

The 10-Meter System determines the path of the Hartmann System (top view). In a side wall of the 10-Meter System, a side wall of the Hartmann System runs as well.

Measuring the Geo-Sha in the Side Walls of the 10-Meter System with the L-Rod, Tensor, and Pendulum

For the **10-Meter System**, proceed in a way similar to that described for the Hartmann System or the 170-Meter System When using the L-rod, ask the question: "*Is a side wall of the 10-Meter System with Geo-Sha here?*" The question to ask with the tensor or pendulum is: "*Are carriers that conduct Geo-Sha into the side walls of the 10-Meter System here?*" or, in the short form: "*Is Geo-Sha of the 10-Meter System here?*" In the process, continue to mentally concentrate on the carrier. If you along search for the side wall of the 10-Meter System without tuning in to a side wall with Geo-Sha, you may find an additional 10-Meter System that does not conduct Geo-Sha. It would then have no significance here. The side wall of the 10-Meter System without Geo-Sha is located approximately in the center between the side walls of the 10-Meter System with Geo-Sha.

The maximum intensity of the Geo-Sha in the side walls of the 10-Meter System varies. The maximum intensity in the walls running in the north-south direction is **60** and **40** in the walls running in an east-west direction. As already described under the watercourses, these values are related to the 2nd level. The intensity of the energy is dependent upon the time of day, the moon cycle, and other factors. We therefore recommend that you also ask about **the maximum night value.**

Hand and Foot Pain Because of Geo-Sha

A feng shui consultant advised an acquaintance at home and at her workplace: "An artist, who successfully made pottery, had pains in her hands that occurred with increasing frequency. At her workplace, I determined a radiation by Geo-Sha. Her workplace was located precisely in a side wall of the 10-Meter System. Just a few days after the sleeping area had been corrected, she was surprised that her hands no longer hurt.

After the workplace renovation, I examined her residence for Geo-Sha and discovered that a side wall of the 10-Meter System ran through the foot end of her bed. She therefore asked me: 'Can it be that my inexplicable foot pains come from this? Up to now, all of the doctors have said I was crazy when I told them that I wake up every morning with foot pain.' After about one week, she called me and proudly announced that her pain had disappeared three days before."

The 250-Meter System

Geo-Sha is conducted from above to below in the side walls of the 250-Meter System as well. The 250-Meter System was first described by Wilhelm Gerstung. It has an average side length and/or average height of approx. 820 feet (250 m). The average side length can fluctuate between about 750 and 890 feet (230 to 270 m). The thickness of the side walls is 20 to 35 inches (50 to 90 cm).

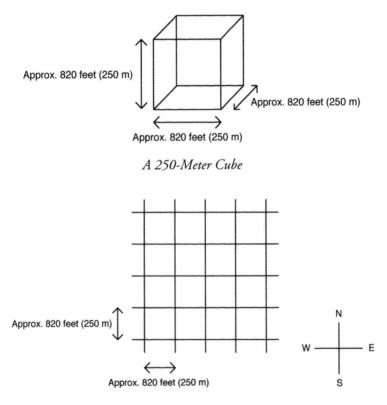

Approx. 820 feet (250 m)

Approx. 820 feet (250 m)

Approx. 820 feet (250 m)

A 250-Meter Cube

Approx. 820 feet (250 m)

Approx. 820 feet (250 m)

N

W ——— E

S

A 250-Meter System (top view).
The distance between the side walls is approx. 820 feet
(750 to 890 ft.) or 250 meters (230 to 270 m).

For the sake of simplicity, we have spoken of one 250-Meter System up to now. However, there are three 250-Meter Systems that have similar characteristics. When you ask your questions, you will therefore also equally find all three systems. This means that you will find two additional 250-Meter Systems between the two side walls of one 250-Meter System. However, these will not be evenly distributed throughout this distance. Two 250-Meter Systems are arranged in such a way that the distance of their side walls from each other is approximately equal in size, which is about 410 feet. In individual cases, the side walls of the third 250-Meter System may also be quite close to one of the side walls of one of the other two 250-Meter Systems.

Measuring the Geo-Sha in the Side Walls of the 250-Meter System with the L-Rod, Tensor, and Pendulum

The question to ask for the L-rod is: *"Is a side wall of the 250-Meter System here?"* The question with the tensor or pendulum is: *"Are carriers that conduct Geo-Sha into the side walls of a 250-Meter System here?"* or, in short form: *"Is Geo-Sha in a 250-Meter System here?"* Continue to concentrate on the carrier while you ask the question. The maximum intensity of Geo-Sha in the side walls of the 250-Meter System is 60. It only reaches 100 in the north-south side wall of the third 250-Meter System mentioned above. These values are related to the 2nd level.

If you have found no 250-Meter System in your house but still want to search for the closest 250-Meter System, you can simplify the search by using the L-rod, for example. Hold *one* L-rod loosely in your right hand and ask: *"In which direction is the closest 250-Meter System?"* The L-rod will then turn in your hand so that it shows the direction in which you can find the closest 250-Meter System. Please be patient and wait until the L-rod has completed its movement and remains calm in your hand. You can naturally also search for the closest watercourse of relevant intensity or a different cube system in the same way. In this manner, you can also determine the direction of north when you don't have a compass or the appropriate map showing the direction of north. If you would like to determine the direction of north in this manner, the best approach is to practice first with the help of a compass or a map.

Waking Up Between Two and Five in the Morning

"Mr. K was advised by his physician to have his home checked by a feng shui expert. During my visit, Mr. K. explained that he had become a nervous wreck. He could not sleep at night between three and five o'clock, then had to get up and read something. Since he had to be up at 6 a.m. to go to work, it practically was not worth going back to bed again.

He slept with his head in a side wall of the 250-Meter System. Since the planned renovation could not be carried out immediately, I recommended that he sleep with his head at the foot of the bed in the meantime. After one week, he called and reported that he already slept much better during the first night. He was still up between four and five a.m., but although he woke up around four a.m. the second night, he did not get up. The third night, he slept throughout the night. As this success continued, he became increasingly calm with time."

Use the L-Rod, Tensor, or Pendulum to Look for Trans-Sha that Has Been Activated by Metals

Now you have learned to find the side walls of the 10-Meter System and 250-Meter System. When metals, as described above, are placed in these side walls, the lenses also accelerate Trans-Sha into the 3rd dimension.

Remember that the form of metal directs Trans-Sha in a certain direction; for example, through points or projecting pieces. Also pay attention to the arc-shape moving downward for longer distances. When Trans-Sha meets further metal parts, the above-mentioned ping-pong effect can occur.

Hold your pair of L-rods, tensor, or pendulum in the imagined extension of the emanation of the tip or projecting parts. Ask: *"Are carriers with Trans-Sha that have been activated because of metal here?"* At both sides of this main direction (a) there is an angle of almost 45 degrees of a secondary direction (b) that is also horizontal. The intensity of the Trans-Sha in the secondary direction is approx. half the intensity of the main direction. Also look for the secondary directions. In addition, a part of the Trans-Sha continues to run horizontally in the cube wall (c).

Side wall
of the cube system

Metal

View from above

Measurement of Trans-Sha that has been activated because of metal in the side wall of a cube system (explanation in text)

Measure the Intensity of Trans-Sha that Has Been Activated Because of Metal

For Trans-Sha that has been activated because of metal, the health-related level is the **1st level**. On the 1st level, we find the following maximum value:
- In the side wall of the 10-Meter System: 50
- In the side wall of the 250-Meter System: 60
- (In the side wall of the Hartmann System or 170-Meter System: 30).

Be sure to mentally concentrate on the 1st level when determining the intensity of the Trans-Sha because of metals. The question could be: *"Is the intensity of the Trans-Sha that has been activated because of metals 5 or above on the 1st level?"* Increase the numerical value, as described in the section on swirling water.

Moon Stripes

Moon stripes are part of an interior structure of a direction-dependent cube system. Moon stripes can have a) an unfavorable influence on our health through Geo-Sha, they can have b) an emotionally unfavorable effect and/or trigger a certain restlessness, or c) they can have a neutral effect on us. However, we will find one of these three possibilities in the same place at a certain point in time.

Geo-Sha in Moon Stripes

The moon stripes run from north-south and east-west. Moon stripes appear like a vertical wall, although they actually consist of pipe-shaped individual structures lined up very closely together. These pipes run at a slight slant in the "wall," whereby the wall itself rises vertically. You will usually find moon stripes in groups, meaning a number of them lined up next to each other. The distance between the individual stripes can be about one to three meters and up to seven stripes can be next to each other. The distance between the stripes occurring in groups is about the same within the individual group.

In terms of health, the effect of Geo-Sha in the moon stripes on human beings is comparable with the effect of Geo-Sha in the 250-Meter System. When the moon is full, the values are distinctly higher than during the new moon. The intensity of Geo-Sha on the

2nd level is maximum of 45 during the full moon and a maximum of 15 during the new moon. These values are valid for the moon stripes that run north-south and those that run east-west.

A Little Girl with Neurodermatitis

A 2 1/2-year-old little girl suffered from neurodermatitis. The symptoms worsened on a regular basis during full moon. A feng shui consultant was contacted and he discovered that a moon stripe with Geo-Sha ran through the child's bed. About 5 weeks after the sleeping area had been corrected, the little girl's complaints improved considerably.

Moon Strips with an Emotionally Unfavorable Effect and Neutral Moon Stripes

Neutral moon stripes can remain neutral in their effects on people for many years and then suddenly show an impact caused by Geo-Sha or an emotionally unfavorable effect. However, the impact of the Geo-Sha and the emotionally unfavorable effect will then usually alternate at short intervals.

Since there are two disruptive types of moon stripes, it is advisable to search for them separately with two subsequent questions. Ask with the L-rod, tensor, or pendulum: *"Is the structure of pipe-like moon stripes with Geo-Sha here?"* and then: *"Is the structure of pipe-like moon stripes that trigger restlessness here?"*

Disruptive Influences Coming Directly from the Side Walls of Direction-Dependent Cube Systems

In the side walls of direction-dependent cube systems, we find a negative impact caused not only by Geo-Sha and Trans-Sha and minimal values for Vital-Qi: The structure itself can exert a disruptive influence.

The 10-Meter System

The structure of a 10-meter side wall can have a particularly negative impact on a human being when the sleeping area is located in the side wall of this system. Both the external aura structure (hull and chakras), as well as the inner aura structure of the human being (for example, the inner meridian system) can be damaged or impaired in their function.

This can especially lead to a limitation in the effects of alternative therapies such as acupuncture, homeopathy, and Bach Flowers, as well as bioresonance therapy. This reaction can even extend to resistance to therapy. False reactions and overreactions can be observed more frequently in these situations. We also recommend not permanently storing things like homeopathic remedies and Bach Flowers in a side wall, especially of the 10-Meter System.

Disruptive Influences Coming Directly from the Structures Above Watercourses and Fault Zones

When building corners from the outside point to a house or a room, the Chinese call these Secret Arrows (*An Jian*). If a room is located directly at the outer wall to which a Secret Arrow points, and if there is an underground watercourse or a fault zone beneath the room, this can have a special activating effect on the structure above the watercourse or the fault zone (see section on Per-Sha). The structure above the water course or fault zone can then have a directly disruptive impact in a special way, in addition to the harmful energy above the watercourse (Trans-Sha) or fault zone (Per-Sha). However, for this to occur, it is necessary that the Secret Arrow hits the watercourse or fault zone at somewhat of a right angle (+/– 20 to 25 degrees). The disruptive influences of these structures on human beings are similar to those described for the 10-Meter System).

Additional Problematic Structures

The Curry System

In contrast to the 10-Meter System, the side walls of the Curry System do not conduct any energy that is harmful for human beings. However, the structure of the Curry System can have an impairing impact on the aura structure of a human being.

The Curry System is a direction-dependent cube system, the side walls of which are aligned approximately in the intermediate directions of NE/SW and NW/SE. These are actually two direction-dependent systems so interlocked with each other that they make the impression of being one single system. The Curry System is named after the German-American Dr. M. Curry, M.D., who based his work on that of the German engineer Siegfried Wittmann.

The average length of the side walls for both systems is approximately 24 feet (19 to 26 ft.) or 7.5 meters (5.9 to 7.8 m) so that a distance of about 12 feet (9 1/2 to 13 ft.) or 3.75 meters (2.95 to 3.9 m) can be found as a result of the interlocking of one side wall.

In addition to the disruptive effect through the structure of the Curry System, which has already been described, the Curry System can also impair sleep by triggering inner restlessness. This additional effect applies to about every third side wall of the Curry System.

You can search for the Curry System by using the following question: *"Is the structure of a Curry System that disturbs the human aura here?"* This question is suitable for searching with the L-rod, the tensor, or the pendulum.

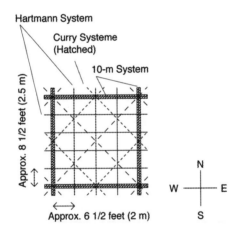

The Curry System (top view).
The intersections of the Curry System, which are located close to the intersection of the 10-Meter System, (almost) correspond with them (Curry System has broken lines).

The 400-Meter System

The structure of the 400-Meter System complex is a special case. The 400-Meter System complex was first described by Jens Mehlhase. Here we find secondary walls parallel to a middle wall (called the main wall) on both sides at a distance of about 60 feet (18 m). These secondary walls are narrower than the main wall. However, the problems described below occur not only in the main wall or the two secondary walls, but also in the entire area between the main wall and the secondary walls. So the width of the entire structure, within which we observe the problems, consists of approx. 120 feet (36 m). The distance from one main wall to the other is approx. 1300 feet (1150–1450 ft.) or 400 meters (350–440 m).

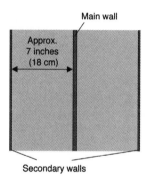

The 400-Meter System complex with the main wall and the two secondary walls.

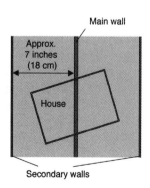

A house in the 400-Meter System complex.

Occupants of a house that stands in the 400-Meter System complex often do not feel very well in their house or apartment, without being able to list any specific reasons for this. Sensitive people frequently feel themselves to be disturbed in quite a direct way, especially at night. It isn't unusual for them to even see demons and distorted faces walking through their room. Even during the daytime, these people may feel extremely ill at ease. People who are less sensitive often feel emotionally affected. They feel more irritable, tend toward depressive moods, and are less concentrated. Problems with disinclination toward work are intensified.

These phenomena can even occur when the afflicted person doesn't even sleep in the main or secondary wall of the 400-Meter System complex but the residence simply has the 400-Meter System complex running through it. The problems can be considerably intensified when the bed of the afflicted person is located in the secondary or especially in the main wall of the 400-Meter System complex. Women and children are more frequently affected than men. Women are also particularly affected to an intensified degree when the southwest corner has been left out of L-shaped houses and is used as a terrace, for example.

You can search for the 400-Meter System complex in the following manner. Ask this question with the L-rod, tensor, or pendulum: *"Is a main or secondary wall of the 400-Meter System complex here?"* When you have found a wall, clarify the situation by asking: "Is the main wall of the 400-Meter System complex here?" If you get a YES, then ask on both sides of the main wall you have found to be sure: *"Am I in the structure of the 400-Meter System complex?"* You must receive a YES on both sides since the structure of the 400-Meter System complex extends out to the secondary wall on both sides of the main wall. If you receive an answer of NO to the question about the main wall, as verification you can ask: *"Is a secondary wall of the 400-Meter System complex here?"* You should now receive a YES. Ask on both sides of the secondary wall that you have found: *"Am I in the structure of the 400-Meter System complex?"* You should only receive a YES on one side of the secondary wall (except if you find yourself at a point where two systems cross). You can look for the main wall at a distance of about 60 feet (18 m) from this side.

A Boy Wakes Up with Nightmares on a Recurrent Basis

An 8-year-old boy frequently came into his parent's bedroom at night because he was plagued by nightmares. As a result, the mother called a friend who was a feng shui consultant. It turned out that the main wall of the 400-Meter System complex ran through the boy's bed. The feng shui consultant advised the mother to place a Feng Shui Power Disc in the house, among other things. A few weeks later, the mother reported that the boy could once again sleep well throughout the night.

Additional Disruptive Influences through Substructures of Direction-Dependent Cube Systems

In addition to the above-described disruptive influences in the side walls of direction-dependent structures, there may also be additional disruptive zones that can be perceived in the form of points or circles. These are various substructures of different direction-dependent cube systems. In general, these are column-like vertical structures with varying diameters. The disruptive influences can either relate to health or have a negative impact on the emotions—or a combination of both.

Typical Health Disorders

If we want to protect our health, it is particularly important to protect ourselves against Geo-Sha and Trans-Sha while we sleep. The impact of these energies during our sleep can trigger a great variety of illnesses and feelings of poor health.

Feelings of Poor Health

Many people experience the effect of these energies in the form of difficulties in falling asleep and sleeping through the night, exhaustion in the morning, or waking up with headache and joint pain. Waking up on a regular basis between 2 and 5 a.m. can also indicate a disturbed sleeping environment.

Chronic Illnesses

Depending upon the body's power of resistance, these energies (particularly in the sleeping area) can also cause chronic diseases to develop over months and years, in addition to disturbances of well-being after having an impact for a longer period of time. Among these are, for example, chronically recurring infections of the upper air passages and rheumatic diseases. Many chronic illnesses can be aided in their development and/or in their manifestation.

This applies in particular to: high blood pressure, diabetes mellitus, diseases of the thyroid gland, chronic women's diseases, allergies, bronchial asthma, neurodermatitis (particularly in children), and chronic skin diseases. Here we find changes for the worse from vein diseases to thrombosis.

Special Impacts on Children

Among other things, the ways that children suffer ranges from babies crying for no known reason and bed-wetting to learning difficulties and concentration problems.

Cancer Diseases and Cardiac Infarction

Particularly worth mentioning is that more than 80 percent of people suffering from **cancer** are affected by Geo-Sha or Trans-Sha from the side walls of the **10-Meter System**. Cancer diseases, in terms of Geo-Sha, are more frequently found in people who sleep in the side walls that run north-south. People who sleep in the side walls that run east-west have a conspicuous frequency of **cardiac infarctions**. This differentiation of the frequency of cancer and cardiac infarctions does not apply to the Trans-Sha that has been activated because of metals in the side walls of the 10-Meter System. For both cancer and cardiac infarction, we find an increased number of diseases here. Trans-Sha that has been activated because of metals in the side walls of the 250-Meter System can also promote the development of cancer diseases.

Overview: Typical Health Disorders through Geo-Sha and Trans-Sha

Feelings of Ill Health
- Difficulties in fall asleep and sleeping through the night
- Tiredness in the morning or waking up with headache or joint pain
- Waking up between 2 and 5 a.m. on a regular basis

Chronic Illnesses
- Chronically returning infections of the upper respiratory tract
- Rheumatic illnesses
- High blood pressure

- Diabetes mellitus
- Diseases of the thyroid gland
- Chronic gynecological disorders
- Allergies
- Bronchial asthma
- Neurodermatitis (especially in children)
- Chronic skin diseases
- Intensification of vein ailments, up to thrombosis

Special Impact on Children
- Babies crying for no apparent reason
- Bedwetting
- Learning difficulties and concentration disorders

The Effects of Geo-Sha and Trans-Sha on the Various Levels

We first want to give an overview of the effects of Geo-Sha and Trans-Sha on the different levels:

Level	*Effects*	*Notes*
1st level	Fostering or development of the above-mentioned illnesses in combination with the finer levels of Geo-Sha and Trans-Sha.	Rare in nature, but frequently occurring because of the use of metal in home construction and decoration (in the form of Trans-Sha).
2nd to 4th level	The effects correspond to those of the 1st level.	Particularly in the side walls of the 10-Meter and 250-Meter System.
5th and 6th level	Sleep disorders, discomfort, exhaustion and tiredness, emotional disorders.	
7th and 8th level	Weakening of the immune system*, thereby fostering the development of illnesses and delays in healing. Intensification of the effects of the Geo-Sha and Trans-Sha on the 1st to 6th levels.	

---

* We understand defense to also include the defensive functions of the immune system, as well as those of our aura.

9th and 10th level	Intensification of the effect on the 1st to 4th level through weakening of the immune system.	Trans-Sha above watercourses and in the side walls of the Hartmann and 170-Meter System are not found on the levels 9 to 12.
11th and 12th level	Lack of drive, depressive bad mood.	See 9th and 10th level

The Interaction of Geo-Sha and Trans-Sha through Metal in the 10-Meter System

The combination of the Geo-Sha and Trans-Sha (through metals) of the various levels is responsible, among other things, for the fact that people with their sleeping area in the side walls of the **10-Meter System** practically have all the illnesses mentioned at the beginning.

Lack of Vital-Qi in Combination with Strain of Geo-Sha and Trans-Sha through Metals

The effect of the strain of Geo-Sha and Trans-Sha through metals is further intensified since there are critically minor values for Vital-Qi found in the side walls of the 10-Meter System. (The significance of Vital-Qi is discussed in *Qi* on page 107 ff.) The interaction of the strain caused by Geo-Sha and Trans-Sha through metals on the various subtle levels on the one hand and the lack of Vital-Qi on the other hand, especially fosters the occurrence of cardiac infarctions and cancer diseases.

Disruptive Influences of the Side-Wall Structure of the 10-Meter System

In addition to the combination of the above-described Geo-Sha or Trans-Sha through metals with a lack of Vital-Qi, there are also other disruptive influences of the structure (also see above) of the side wall of the 10-Meter System itself. These combinations of three in the side wall of the 10-Meter System ultimately lead to the serious illnesses described above.

At the same time, we should not overlook the fact that the constitution of the patient is very important in assessing the seriousness of the illness and time period during which the person in the sleeping area was exposed to the energies until the illness breaks out. Furthermore, genetic factors, nutrition, and emotional influences also play an important role, as well as environmental strains and other influences from the person's lifestyle.

Breast Cancer in a Side Wall of the 10-Meter System

The 40-year-old Dagmar M. noticed a palpable knot in her left breast. At first, she refused to believe that it could be something serious. However, the doctors diagnosed it as breast cancer. An operation took place. The left mammary gland was removed; fortunately, the lymph tracts were all in order.

Ms. M. had not smoked or drank excessive alcohol, and she had made an effort to eat a healthy and balanced diet. Yet, she had developed breast cancer. How could this have happened?

Ms. M. knew that her mother and cousins had developed cancer, so that a hereditary predisposition for this disease existed. On the other hand, she also knew many women who had frequent cases of cancer in their families yet themselves remained healthy until a ripe old age. So what could have been the special cause in her case?

A doctor, who was also a friend of hers, did a feng shui examination of her home. The doctor walked through her bedroom with the tensor in his right hand and determined that a side wall of the 10-Meter System ran through her bed, and did so from her right foot to her left shoulder. So Ms. M. was laying directly in the emanating area of the 10-Meter System with her diseased left breast. As a result, the doctor suggested that the bed be moved about one meter to the side. This was done immediately. In addition, the doctor told Ms. M. that she should not place her nightstand lamp in the path of the side walls of the 10-Meter System. The metal from the stand and wire basket of the lampshade would otherwise activate further unfavorable energies, Trans-Sha.

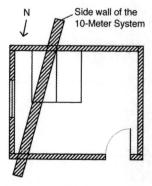

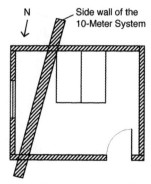

A woman with breast cancer sleeps in one side wall of the 10-Meter System.

The bed was moved.

Effects of the Hartmann and 170-Meter System, as well as Underground Watercourses

With the exception of serious internal diseases such as cancer and cardiac infarction, all of the above-described illnesses and feelings of poor health can be found in the side walls of the Hartmann and 170-Meter System, as well as underground watercourses. The time period that is necessary in order to produce the respective illnesses or disorders is greater here than for the 10-Meter System. Among other things, this is because of the lesser intensity of the energies found here.

Per-Sha

A Further Type of Sha: Per-Sha

Per-Sha is the general term for inauspicious energies that behave differently in the 5th dimension than Trans-Sha or Geo-Sha. We must also ask about them separately with the tensor or pendulum. We initially want to discuss the two types of Per-Sha that we find in fault zones

---

What is Per-Sha?
Per-Sha is a general term for harmful energies in fault zones, clock radios with a red digital display, and satellite dishes.

Per-Sha Above Fault Zones

There are many faults or folds in the earth's crust. Because of the interruption of the even layers, cracks and fissures, an invisible structure is formed above. Similar to the direction-dependent cube wall, in this structure unfavorable energies are accelerated from a higher dimension into the 3rd dimension through an interface. In this case, there are two different energies that come from the 5th dimension. These two energies can be differentiated on the basis of the direction of flow that they have in the 5th dimension. Seen from our dimension, we can state this direction of flow with an angle to the horizon.

Per-Sha 61 and Per-Sha 51

The flow direction of one of the energies has an angle of 61 degrees to the horizontal plane in the 5th dimension (Per-Sha 61); the other's direction of flow is 51 degrees to the horizontal plane (Per-Sha 51). Both energies move in the 3rd dimension from below to above in a slightly fan-shaped form. They have a Yang effect on human beings so that we find special disruptions as health disorders or illnesses, which the Chinese call illnesses with an excess of Yang. (See the beginning of *Qi* page 105 for some comments about yin and yang). Among these are:

Per-Sha 61
• High blood pressure
• Hyperactivity
• Headache (at the side, as well as on top of the cranium)
• Loud voice

Per-Sha 51
• Sleep disorders
• Tendency toward aggravation and anger

Look for Fault Zones!

You can look for fault zones in your room or on your property in a way similar to the method described under the section on watercourses. In the process, ask separate questions for each of the energies mentioned above. When you search with the L-rod, ask: *"Are structures above a fault zone that conduct Per-Sha 61 upward here?"* When you search with the tensor or pendulum, ask: *"Are carriers with Per-Sha 61 above fault zones here?"*

For the L-rod, the question about the latter energy is: *"Are structures above a fault zone that could conduct Per-Sha 51 upward?"* With the tensor or the pendulum, the question is: *"Are carriers with Per-Sha 51 above fault zones here?"*

When you have found a fault zone, determine the intensity of the respective Per-Sha. The maximum intensity of Per-Sha 61 is 30, as for watercourses, and Per-Sha 51 has a maximum intensity of 17, both measured on the 2nd level respectively. Be sure to individually determine the intensity above the part of the fault zone that demonstrates the strongest emanation. You can search for this part with a question like: *"Is the strongest intensity of Per-Sha above this fault zone?"* Cross the fault zone once diagonally while asking this question. If you don't receive a YES because the radiation is unequally distributed in the course of the zone, then it may suffice to ask: *"Is the strongest intensity of the fault zone's Per-Sha that I find in this crossing located here?"* Then measure the intensity.

High Blood Pressure Above a Fault Zone

A 30-year-old man had suffered high blood pressure for the past one-and-a-half years. His face was conspicuously red. He particularly complained about head congestion every morning. During the feng shui examination, it became apparent that his sleeping area was located above a fault zone with a great intensity of Per-Sha. After his sleeping area had been corrected, the symptoms improved after several weeks, accompanied by a simultaneous therapy with the WS Frequency Device.

Per-Sha in the Side Walls of the Hartmann System

If there is a fault zone in the vicinity of the side walls of the Hartmann System, these side walls conduct Per-Sha in an upward direction. This is the same energy as found above the fault zones.

The Effect of Clock Radios with Red Digital Displays

Not only fault zones can accelerate energies that are inauspicious for human beings into our dimension. Clock radios with red digital displays are also capable of this. These are primarily cheap products produced in the Far East. Clock radios with green, bluish, or black displays (in a gray field) do not give off the emanation described above.

Per-Sha 36

A large portion of these clock radios with red digital displays accelerate a further type of Per-Sha from the 5th dimension into the 3rd dimension. In contrast to the energies above fault zones, this is an energy that has a flow direction at the angle of 36 degrees to the horizon in the 5th dimension. We therefore call this energy Per-Sha 36. This energy has an effect on human beings very similar to the effect of Geo-Sha and Trans-Sha. The expansion of this energy into our dimension is practically horizontal, up to 10 meters to the front; it does not go as far toward the back and to the side, and the intensity is less in these directions.

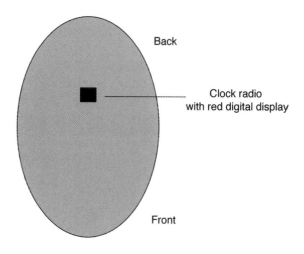

The effective range of Per-Sha that can be activated by a clock radio with a red digital display (top view).

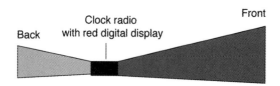

The effective range of Per-Sha that can be activated by a clock radio with a red digital display (cross-section).

In addition to the typical health disorders already mentioned for Geo-Sha, the following are particularly conspicuous in the case of Per-Sha: chronic bronchitis, headaches, shoulder pain, epilepsy-like attacks, facial erysipelas, and tinnitus (ringing in the ears).

A suitable way of asking the question when searching with the L-rod is: *"Is a structure with Per-Sha 36 that has been activated by a clock radio with a red digital display here?"* A suitable question for the tensor or pendulum is: *"Are carriers with Per-Sha 36 that have been activated by a clock radio with a red digital display here?"* The maximum intensity of Per-Sha 36 on the 2nd level is 66; on the 1st level it is 41 (each on a scale of 0 to 100). It is sufficient to determine the intensity of Per-Sha 36 on the 2nd level.

Neck Pain Because of a Clock Radio

A 48-year-old sales employee had pains in his neck that could not be explained by orthodox medicine. He had a feng shui examination done in his apartment. A clock radio with a red digital display was standing on his nightstand. The feng shui consultant advised him to remove the clock radio, which was quickly thrown into the garbage. The pains in the neck completely subsided after a few days.

Clock radios obviously not only cause problems through Per-Sha 36, but can also create a negative impact on the sleeping area in particular because of electrosmog.

Satellite Dishes Can Also Activate Per-Sha

Satellite dishes can also activate Per-Sha. Per-Sha, which is activated through satellite dishes, has various angles to the horizontal plane in the 5th dimension. However, when searching for this with the L-rod, tensor, or pendulum, it suffices to generally ask about the Per-Sha that has been activated by the satellite dishes. The activated Per-Sha moves away from the satellite dish in two directions. On the one hand, it moves diagonally toward the back and downward in the angle at which the satellite dish has been installed. The effect is similar to that of a clock radio with a red digital display. The main effect here is on the 2nd level. On the other hand, it moves horizontally toward the rear and tends to have a negative impact on us in the mental area. The main effect here is on the 9th and 10th level.

A suitable question for searching with the L-rod is: *"Is a structure with Per-Sha that has been activated by a satellite dish here?"* With the tensor or pendulum, you can ask: *"Are carriers with Per-Sha that has been activated by a satellite dish here?"*

At this point, we would like to briefly mention that various types of Per-Sha can be found in the area beneath *diagonal attic windows*. The decisive factor here is the angle of the diagonal attic window to the horizontal plane. We are most likely to find relevant influences on the levels 5 to 7. On these levels, these types of Per-Sha can disturb the well-being and concentration of our mental aspects, among other things.

Overview of Energies and Maximum Values in the Various Disruptive Zones

10-Meter System	*Geo-Sha*, maximum value of 60 on the 2nd level in the side wall that runs north-south, 40 in the side wall that runs east-west	*Trans-Sha through metals*, maximum value of 50 on the 1st level
250-Meter System	*Geo-Sha*, maximum value of 60 on the 2nd wall; only reaches 100 in the side wall running north-south of one of the three 250-Meter Systems	*Trans-Sha through metals*, maximum value of 60 on the 1st level
Moon Stripes	*Geo-Sha*, maximum value of 45 on the 2nd level during full moon, maximum of 15 during new moon	*Trans-Sha through metals*, maximum value of 20 on the 1st level
170-Meter System	*Trans-Sha*, maximum value of 30 on the 2nd level for both 170-Meter Systems	*Trans-Sha through metals*, maximum value of 30 on the 1st level

Watercourses	*Trans-Sha*, maximum value of 30 on the 2nd level	*Trans-Sha through metals*, maximum value of 30 on the 1st level
Hartmann System	*Trans-Sha*, maximum value of 30 on the 2nd level Close to fault zones: *Per-Sha 61* and *Per-Sha 51*, see Fault Zones for maximum value on the 2nd level	*Trans-Sha through metals*, maximum value of 30 on the 1st level
Fault Zones	*Per-Sha 61*, maximum value of 30 on the 2nd level *Per-Sha 51*, maximum value of 17 on the 2nd level	*No Trans-Sha through metals*
Curry System	No Geo-Sha, Trans-Sha, or Per-Sha, but disruptive influence through the structure	
400-Meter System Complex	No Geo-Sha, Trans-Sha, or Per-Sha in relevant intensity, but triggers restlessness, among other things	
Clock Radio with Red Digital Display	*Per-Sha 36*, maximum value of 66 on the 2nd level, maximum value of 41 on the 1st level	
Satellite Dish	*Various types of Per-Sha*, strongest effect in diagonal direction downward and toward the back on the 2nd level, maximum value of 38 (average value of 13-14) on the 2nd level, strongest effect in the horizontal direction toward the back on the 9th and 10th level	

Examining the Sleeping Area for Geo-Sha, Trans-Sha, and Per-Sha

The examination of the sleeping area described here should be done in a particularly careful manner if the problematic structures in the house cannot be corrected through a Feng Shui Power Disc 99 or Tachyonized Silica Discs in a special arrangement (see Chapter 5, on page 121 ff). A thorough examination of the sleeping area can also help clarify whether the sleeping area may have played a role in the development of a health disorder.

What You Should Do Before Actually Examining the Sleeping Area

Before examining the sleeping area, you should get a picture of the surrounding environment. We recommend, if possible, that you walk through the entire house once. While doing so, pay attention to any large metal parts that could conduct Trans-Sha into the house. These may be either movable or permanently installed metal parts. Among the **movable metal parts** that we frequently find are cars, movable trash containers, as well as garage doors. Movable metal parts may lead to changing the course of the side walls of the 10-Meter and 250-Meter systems. Among the **permanently installed metal parts** on the house are balcony railings, metal eaves, gutters, satellite dishes, among other things. In addition, you will possibly find clearly visible sources of strain because of high-tension power lines like long-distance transmission lines, transformer stations, or electrified railroad and streetcar routes (see the section on *Feng Shui and Electrosmog* on page 154 ff).

Examining the Sleeping Area for Geo-Sha and Trans-Sha

When people have already slept in the same sleeping area for several years and health disorders have occurred during this time (as described in the section on *Typical Health Disorders* on page 77 ff, you should search with particular care for a negative impact on the sleeping environment because of Geo-Sha or Trans-Sha.

When examining it, we recommend that you look for the path of the side walls of the **10-Meter and 250-Meter System** in the house or apartment. This is significant since not only a direct strain on the sleeping area may exist, but Trans-Sha can also be conducted into the bedroom through metals. Determine the course of the above-mentioned cube system in the house or apartment with the L-rod, tensor, or pendulum, as described in previous sections.

Take particular care in examining the bedroom for moon stripes, as well as Trans-Sha above underground **watercourses** and in the side walls of **the Hartmann and the 170-Meter System**. You should also look for **fault zones**, the **Curry System**, the **400-Meter System complex**, as well as the **influences of satellite dishes**.

Special Circumstances at Night

When examining the sleeping environment for Geo-Sha and Trans-Sha, remember that the nightly situations in the bedroom are often different from those during the day. Lowered metal blinds and cars that park in front of the house or in the garage during the night can conduct Trans-Sha into the house or shift it into the side walls of the 10-Meter or 250-Meter System. In the process, either an attraction or a rejection may occur in the side walls of the system.

What You Can Do in Case of Doubt

If you have determined that there is a strain on a person because of Geo-Sha, Trans-Sha through metals, Trans-Sha, or Per-Sha (see next section), yet cannot find any negative impact on the sleeping environment, you should search for the source of the strain until you have clearly located it. For example, there may be an intensive strain at the workplace, particularly if the person works in a sitting position. In case of doubt, the examination of the sleeping environment must be repeated during the night if no other explanation can be found for the strain. After the sleeping environment has been corrected and the affected person has engaged in the appropriate therapy, you should once again examine the patient for a strain because of Geo-Sha, Trans-Sha, and Per-Sha.

Diagnosis of the Strain on Human Beings Because of Geo-Sha, Trans-Sha, and Per-Sha

The strain on a human being because of Geo-Sha, Trans-Sha, and Per-Sha can be directly determined by using the tensor, pendulum, or another direct testing method like kinesiology. Even if no strain above the individual threshold value have been determined by using the tensor or pendulum, we recommend that you still place a Feng Shui Power Disc 99 in the house. It may be that the respective person places metal objects in the side wall of the 10-Meter System, for example, at a later point in time and thereby unknowingly creates a strain upon himself or herself.

The Individual Threshold Value

The individual threshold value for a harmful energy indicates how much the individual person can tolerate of this energy on a scale of 0 to 100 maximum without becoming ill. The individual threshold value for Geo-Sha Trans-Sha, and Per-Sha usually lies between 4 and 5.

Measuring Geo-Sha on the Human Being

In order to test a human being, it has proved effective to ask above the head of the respective person with the tensor or pendulum: *"Is this person negatively affected by Geo-Sha that goes beyond his or her individual threshold value?"* Particularly for examinations with the pendulum, the person being examined should sit down so that there is enough space above the head to measure. We recommend that not only the 2nd level be measured, as previously, but that the strain on the 10th level also be taken into account in this overall questioning. In order to be sure, you should additionally ask: *"Is this person strained beyond his or her individual threshold value by Geo-Sha of the 10th level?"*

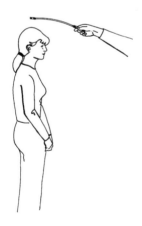

Measurement of Geo-Sha, Trans-Sha, and Per-Sha on the human being (overall questioning above the head of the person).

When you have determined a strain because of Geo-Sha above the individual threshold value on the person, it is useful to proceed in sections directly on the body and ask about the intensity of the strain: *"Is the most intense strain because of Geo-Sha on this person in the head area?"* If this is the case, ask about a strain on the individual head sections. Proceed in a systematic manner, and pay attention to the ears, nose, and mouth. Next, ask at the back, on the front side of the trunk, and on the arms and legs in a similar systematic way. In the process, the strain on the inner organs, such as the liver, gall bladder, stomach, etc., as well as the individual joints, can also be determined.

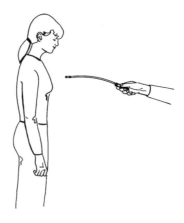

Measurement of Geo-Sha, Trans-Sha, and Per-Sha on the human being. The tensor or pendulum is held in front of the respective body sections.

Determining the Intensity of the Strain

When you have found the region of the body that is most intensely strained, we also recommend that you ask about the intensity of this strain. It is best to measure the intensity of the strain on the 2nd level. The question is: *"Is the intensity of the strain caused by Geo-Sha on this region of the body on the 2nd level 5 or above?"* Increase the numerical value in the same way as above.

Measuring Trans-Sha through Metals and Trans-Sha
on Human Beings

You can basically sue a similar approach to determining the strain caused by Trans-Sha through metals and Trans-Sha. If Trans-Sha through metals is activated in a side wall of the 10-Meter or 250-Meter System, you will find the most intense strain on the 1st level. You should therefore ask: *"Is this person strained beyond his or her individual threshold value on the 1st level?"*

If you want to determine the strain of Trans-Sha above watercourses, as well as in the side walls of the Hartmann and 170-Meter Systems, on human beings, then ask: *"Is this person strained above his or her individual threshold value by Trans-Sha on the 2nd level?"*

When determining the most intensely strained area of the body and the intensity of the strain, use the approach described in previous sections.

Measuring Per-Sha on Human Beings

When asking the following questions, you can attune yourself to the 2nd level. It is best to first find out whether the respective person has a clock radio with a red digital display on the nightstand or somewhere else in the bedroom. If there is such a clock radio in the room, you can determine a possible negative impact using the tensor or pendulum. The question should be:

"Is this person negatively affected by Per-Sha 36 that is above his or her individual threshold value?"

Afterward, ask about a negative impact because of Per-Sha above a fault zone. The best approach is to ask separately about Per-Sha 61 and Per-Sha 51.

"Is this person strained by Per-Sha 61 above his or her individual threshold value?"

"Is this person strained by Per-Sha 51 above his or her individual threshold value?"

When there is a satellite dish on or on top of the house, also ask: *"Is this person strained above his or her individual threshold value by the Per-Sha on the 2nd level that is activated by satellite dishes?"* This type of Per-Sha moves down and to the back in a diagonal direction from the satellite dish. Also ask about a strain on the 6th level: *"Is this person strained above his or her individual threshold value by the Per-Sha on the 6th level that is activated by satellite dishes?"* This type of Per-Sha moves to the back on the horizontal plane. In this case, it is simpler for you to ask about a strain on the 6th level on human beings than about a strain on the 9th and 10th level.

Therapy of the Strain Because of Geo-Sha, Trans-Sha, and Per-Sha

If no therapy of the strain because of Geo-Sha, Trans-Sha through metals, Trans-Sha, and Per-Sha is carried out, the spontaneous reduction of the strain may take several months or years. Children and people with a good defensive condition can usually recover rather quickly from these types of strain. Older people and those who generally have a weaker defense system often require additional therapy.*

Reduction of Strain Because of Geo-Sha, Trans-Sha, and Per-Sha with the WS Frequency Device

For many years now, the WS Frequency Spectrum Effect Physiatrics Apparatus—called **WS Frequency Device** here—has proved to be effective (see Information and Advise in appendix for supply sources). WS stands for "wide spectrum." The device was developed in China in the middle of the 1980s and employs the healing effect of selected natural stones, of which people have known for thousands of years. The stone powder is applied to the ceramic rods, which have been heated electrically. It supports the human immune system by having an effect on a human being's aura. The device creates a frequency spectrum that is very similar to that of the human aura: a resonance vibration occurs. Since the frequency spectrum is set up to be very wide, the WS Frequency Device can be successfully employed for many health disorders. Increasingly more physicians and healing practitioners are now using the WS Frequency Device to reduce the strain existing in the body and the aura caused by Geo-Sha, Trans-Sha through metals, Trans-Sha, and Per-Sha—after the sleeping area has been successfully corrected—down to the individual threshold value.

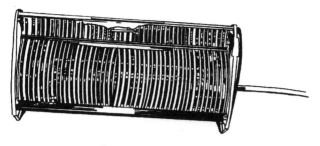

The WS Frequency Device

Energetic "Openings" Increase the Success of the Therapy

It is not absolutely necessary to do the energetic openings described in the following before each treatment. However, they can accelerate the reduction of the strain because of Geo-Sha, Trans-Sha through metals, Trans-Sha, and Per-Sha. In addition, slight physical reactions (light congestion of the head or short-term palpitations of the heart) can be avoided. However, they should be carried out in any case when such physical reactions have occurred.

Energetic Opening of the Feet and Hands

Before you begin the treatment, you should energetically open the **feet** and **hands** of the patient. Stand facing the patient. Hold his or her left foot with your right hand and his or her right foot with your left hand. Place the thumb of each hand onto the instep and the rest of the fingers onto the center of the sole (arch of the foot). In general, you will now feel a flow of energy. You may sense this as tingling, a sense of warmth, a cold feeling, a slight twinge, or light pressure. If you feel nothing like this, ask if the patient has felt something (this will usually be the case). Even if neither you nor the patient has felt something, it can be assumed that an energetic opening has taken place. Leave your hands in this position for about one minute. Do the same thing with the patient's hands. You can either have your thumb on the outside surface of the hands or the palms since this is irrelevant for the energetic opening of the hands. You and/or the patient will feel the energies in the opening of the hands in a manner exactly the same as or similar to how it occurred with the feet.

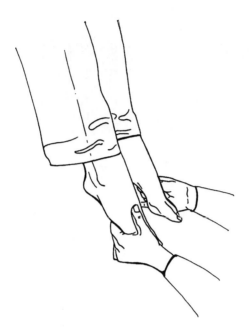

Energetic opening of the feet

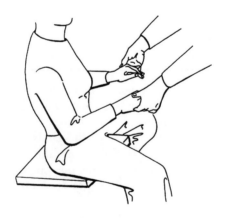

Energetic opening of the hands

Additional Energetic Openings

We recommend that you do further energetic openings using the WS Frequency Device. Stand sideways to the right or left next to the patient. With the three middle fingers of one hand, touch the **lower tip of the breastbone** while touching **the spinal column at the same height on the opposite side** with the three middle fingers of the other hand. You will perceive an energetic opening, similar to that of the feet and hands. This opening can be particularly recommended when the patient suffers from heart trouble.

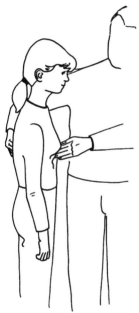

Energetic opening between the lower tip of the breastbone and the spinal column at the same height on the other side.

Both of the following energetic openings can be particularly recommended when the region of the body suffering from the emanations is in the head area. These openings should also be done for people who complain of headaches or slight congestion in the head. Once again, stand to the side of the patient. Place the middle or index finger of one hand **above the indentation of the larynx** and the three middle fingers of the other hand on the **vertex of the head.** Your perception of the energies will again be similar to that described above.

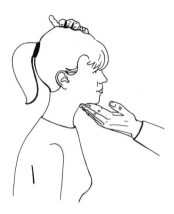

Energetic opening above the indentation of the larynx and the vertex of the head

You should also stand to the side of the patient for the second energetic head opening. Place one to three fingers of the one hand lightly on the **forehead chakra** (in the middle between the eyebrows) and the three middle fingers of the other hand on the **occipital bone on the head** (back of the head). After this last energetic opening, begin with the treatment.

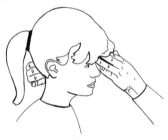

Energetic opening between the forehead chakra and the occipital bone (back of the head)

Use of the WS Frequency Device

The WS Frequency Device is placed 8 to 15 inches (20 to 40 cm) in front of the region of the body strained by Geo-Sha, Trans-Sha through metals, Trans-Sha, and Per-Sha. First turn the device to the level LOW; after 3 to 5 minutes turn it on high. We recommend that you hold the tensor or pendulum between the WS Frequency Device and the negatively affected region of the body. Mental concentration on certain wavelengths is not necessary in this case. In the process, varying movement patterns may occur. Move the tensor or pendulum until the required treatment has been completed.

The strain because of Geo-Sha, Trans-Sha through metals, Trans-Sha, and Per-Sha is already considerably reduced after just one treatment. You can ascertain this by determining the current strain value with the tensor or pendulum, as described above, before the treatment. Then compare this with the strain value that you determine immediately after the treatment. The strain value will increase again somewhat the next day; however, it will still be considerably less than the value you determined before the treatment. A number of treatments are generally necessary in order to come down to or below the individual threshold value.

The best approach is to determine the length of time for the individual applications with the tensor or pendulum. We recommend that you determine the current strain value with the tensor or pendulum each time before and after the application. The frequency of the application should be oriented upon the values that you have determined.

The WS Frequency Device can also be employed without using the tensor or pendulum. In this case, we recommend that the patient be seated with the strained body regions in front of the WS Frequency Device for about 45 minutes during the first application; 30 minutes are adequate for the second time. For further applications, 20 or 15 minutes are recommended. In general, five applications are sufficient against strain because of Geo-Sha, Trans-Sha through metals, Trans-Sha, and Per-Sha.

Polyxans

One suitable alternative in the therapy for strain because of Geo-Sha, Trans-Sha through metals, Trans-Sha, and Per-Sha are the so-called polyxans made by the Ritsert company*. The polyxans are homeopathic potency accords of Carex flava, elong., and vesic. from geobiologically varied growth zones. The specialties **Polyxan Green Comp. Drops** (Polyxan gruen comp. Tropfen), **Polyxan Blue Comp. Drops** (Polyxan blau comp. Tropfen), and **Polyxan Yellow Comp. Drops** (Polyxan gelb comp. Tropfen) are available in bottles

---

* Available in international drugstores.

of 30 milliliters each. The Polyxan Green Comp. is suitable as therapy for the balanced reaction type; Polyxan Blue Comp. for the yang reaction type; and Polyxan Yellow Comp. for the yin reaction type. The normal dosage is 3 x 8 drops, whereby the use of a 30-milliliter bottle is frequently adequate for the length of the application. Both the type of remedy and its dosage and length of use should be checked by using the tensor or pendulum.

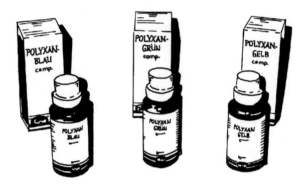

Polyxans

Determining the Appropriate Polyxans

There are two possibilities for determining the suitable polyxans.:
1) Put the respective polyxan in the hand of the person who has been negatively affected and ask the questions formulated below. The tensor or pendulum will give you the familiar reactions for YES or NO.
2) A second possibility is to place the respective polyxan on a table. The person who has been negatively affected lays his or her opened hand on the table at a distance of about 12–15 inches (30 to 40 cm) away from the polyxan. The palm of the hand faces the polyxan while doing so. Hold your tensor or pendulum between the palm of the hand and the polyxan, then ask the questions formulated below. You will get a different response from the tensor or pendulum in this relationship test. If the polyxan is suitable (the answer YES), the tensor or pendulum will move back and forth between the palms of the hands and polyxan. If the polyxan is unsuitable (the answer NO), the tensor will move up

and down. The pendulum turns at a 90-degree angle for the YES reaction. We could say it cuts through the relationship between the polyxan and the person's hand.

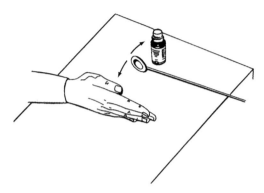

YES reaction of the tensor in the polyxan test

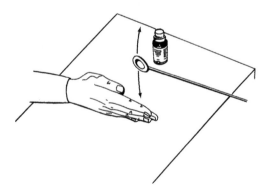

NO reaction of the tensor in the polyxan test (whether the ring of the tensor is held vertically or horizontally is insignificant in terms of the reaction).

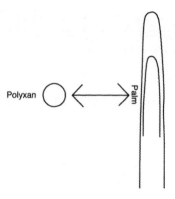

YES reaction of the pendulum in the polyxan test (viewed from above).

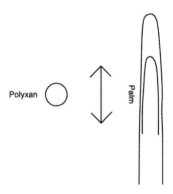

NO reaction of the pendulum in the polyxan test (viewed from above).

Asking the Question for the Right Polyxan

For strain because of Geo-Sha, Trans-Sha through metals, Trans-Sha, and Per-Sha, the suitable polyxan should be determined separately with the tensor or pendulum. When there is a strain because of **Geo-Sha**, the appropriate question to ask is: *"Is polyxan ... (description) best suited for ... (name of person) to eliminate the strain because of Geo-Sha?"* Ask about the three polyxans, one after the other. You will generally receive just one YES.

If there is strain because of *Trans-Sha through metals*, ask: *"Is polyxan ... (description) best suited for ... (name of person) to eliminate the strain because of Trans-Sha through metals?"* It may be here that you receive a YES for Polyxan Yellow and Polyxan Green. This means that a combination therapy with Polyxan Yellow and Green would be best suited for the person strained by Trans-Sha through metals.

If there is strain because of **Trans-Sha** (above watercourses or from the Hartmann or 170-Meter System), ask: *"Is polyxan ... best suited for ... (name of person) to eliminate the strain because of Trans-Sha through metals?"* You will usually receive a YES for Polyxan Yellow or Green.

When you ask about the most suitable polyxan for strain because of **Per-Sha**, you will mainly find Polyxan Blue Comp. You will most likely find Polyxan Green Comp. when there is a mixed strain, but Polyxan Yellow Comp. is extremely rare. Word your question in a way similar to those above.

If there is a strain simultaneously because of Geo-Sha, Trans-Sha through metals, Trans-Sha, and/or Per-Sha, you will not find more than two different polyxans to be suitable. You will only find the combination of Polyxan Yellow with Polyxan Green here. Polyxan Blue is practically only found as an individual medication.

If you have determined just one polyxan, also find the number of days for which the respective person should take the polyxan in the customary dosage of 3 x 8 drops. Ask: *"Should ... (name of person) take Polyxan (description) for five days or longer?"* Go through the number of days one by one until you receive a NO. The last question to which you have received a YES gives you the right amount of days.

If you have determined two polyxans, you must find out how often the respective polyxan should be taken each day. In the process, you will find out that one polyxan should be taken once a day and the second polyxan should be taken twice a day. Have the patient take the polyxan that should be taken once a day at noon and the other morning and night.

Chapter 4

Qi

Positive Energies

The Chinese call the energies that are positive for human beings Qi and Shen, among other things. They have created a variety of sub-terms for Qi, but we do not want to use them here since they may be more confusing than helpful for the Western reader. The different energies that are positive for human beings are subject to various laws. The Analytical School differentiates between these energies according to their behavior in the 5th dimension. This helps in finding **Perm-Qi, Vital-Qi**, and **Shen**, among other energies, with the tensor or pendulum. In Chapter 8, on page 175 ff we will discuss Shen in the section on *Trigram Sectors Can Influence Your Health*. These positive energies can also be differentiated according to yin and yang.

Yin and Yang

The Chinese says that everything has two sides: Yin and Yang. **Yang** stands for: masculine, light, strong, active, forwards, outside, high, full, pointed, hot, dry, new, for the day, and for life. **Yin** represents: feminine, dark, weak, passive, backwards, inside, low, empty, round, cold, moist, old, for the night, and for death. These qualities do not mean a valuation according to good and bad. Instead, the Chinese strive for a balanced state of Yin and Yang. Among other things, they classify illnesses according to this system of whether there is an excess or lack of yin or yang.

Vital-Qi

What is Vital-Qi?
Vital-Qi is an energy that is positive for human beings. It is a type of Qi and important for the vital functions and the defensive function of the immune system.

Vital-Qi is important for the vital functions and the defensive functions of our immune system. The Chinese give the name of **Wei-Qi** to Vital-Qi within the human body. We absorb Vital-Qi through our aura, our respiration, and our food. We absorb both yang Vital-Qi and yin Vital-Qi. Dependent upon whether the deficiency tends to be more yang Vital-Qi or yin Vital-Qi, the following symptoms and complaints may occur, among other things:

A) Deficiency of Yang Vital-Qi:
- Fatigue, as from oppressive air
- Old wounds break open and bleed again
- Absentmindedness, sullenness
- Pains in previously injured body parts when weather changes
- Chest complaints
- Cardiac irregularity
- Ravenous hunger, but quickly satisfied
- Shooting pains, spasmodic contractions, rumbling in entire abdominal area
- Sterility
- Menstruation too early
- Menstruation too long and too intense
- Pain in the ankles
- Pain in the corns
- Pain in the toe nails, as if ingrown
- Feeling as if tendons in hollow of knee are too short
- Infectious disorders and nutritive disturbances on the hands and in the joints
- Epithelial abnormalities of growth (psoriasis)
- Feeling of coldness throughout entire body, even in warm rooms
- Shivering
- Difficulty sleeping through the night without waking up, with deep sleep toward the morning

- General lowered resistance with recurring colds and itching of the skin may also have a deficiency of yang Vital-Qi as a contributing factor.

b) Deficiency of Yin Vital-Qi:
- Sleepiness during the day
- Old wounds break open and bleed again
- Cancer
- Facial hyperidrosis (sweating) without heat
- Feeling of heat throughout entire body with cold hands and/or feet
- Feeling as if a draft is passing over the body or individual parts of the body
- Restless sleep with talking, singing, and snoring
- Sleeping on the back with one hand beneath the head

Absorbable Vital-Qi Is Important for Human Beings

One type of Vital-Qi can be absorbed by human beings, but the other type cannot be absorbed by human beings. Vital-Qi can always be found as yang Vital-Qi and yin Vital-Qi. Since the values for yin Vital-Qi are generally lower than the values for yang Vital-Qi, it is advisable to only determine the values for yin Vital-Qi, meaning absorbable yin Vital-Qi. When we state the values for Vital-Qi in the following text, we mean the values for absorbable yin Vital-Qi. The determination of intensity of Vital-Qi and other positive energies results on a scale of 0 to 100. The value of 100 indicates the highest possible value here. However, this value is usually never achieved in practical terms. For other positive energies as well, it is best to only determine the intensity of the absorbable portion of the respective energy.

Without the use of feng shui remedies, a person can absorb Vital-Qi (absorbable Vital-Qi) at a maximum level of 12, even if there were more in the room. At night, a healthy person requires Vital-Qi with a value of at least 10. On the other hand, ill or older people tend to need Vital-Qi with a value of 12. Vital-Qi values below 2 pose a critical situation for a person's health, especially when there is an additional strain because of Geo-Sha or Trans-Sha through metals. We can find such values in the side walls of the 10-Meter System, for example

Loss of Vital-Qi through Metals

There is generally enough Vital-Qi present in a natural setting. The value for absorbable (yin) Vital-Qi is ordinarily around 10 to 11, although it is often just 7 in full sunlight. In **closed rooms**, Vital-Qi enters together with the air. If there was a house with absolutely no metals in it, the Vital-Qi value would be about 7.

When metals are located in the side walls of the **10-Meter** or **250-Meter System**, which means that Trans-Sha through metals develops, the result is an almost total loss of Vital-Qi in the room. The Vital-Qi that was previously bound to the air then disappears into a higher dimension after a short amount of time. Only values of 1 or just above 1 can be found. Metals in the side walls of the Hartmann or 170-Meter System, as well as those above watercourses, have a similar but lesser effect. Then we frequently find values of just 2 to 3 in the room.

Running underfloor heating made of copper or steel pipes also leads to a disappearance of Vital-Qi. The values for Vital-Qi in the room are then just 3 to 4.

Loss of Vital-Qi through Metals in the Adjoining Room

Take into consideration that in individual cases metals in an adjoining room can also reduce the Vital-Qi in the bedroom, even if Trans-Sha does not penetrate the room walls. In these cases, the carrier of the Trans-Sha comes through the wall room without the energy itself. You can recognize this with the tensor or pendulum when you ask about the carrier of the Trans-Sha without the energy itself: *"Are carriers without Trans-Sha that reduce the Vital-Qi coming from the adjoining room to a relevant degree?"*

Loss of Vital-Qi through High Tension

In the section on *Feng Shui and Electrosmog* on page 154 ff we point out that electromagnetic fields also have an influence on subtle energies. The important factor here is the influence on Vital-Qi, among other things. In the vicinity of high-tension power lines and railway power facilities, we find a distinct reduction of Vital-Qi within a radius of up to 40 meters.

Measure Absorbable Yin Vital-Qi with the Tensor or Pendulum!

Now that you have read about Vital-Qi, you will certainly be interest to know how you can measure the absorbable yin Vital-Qi with the tensor or pendulum.

Measuring the Intensity of Absorbable Yin Vital-Qi

Ask: *"Is the intensity of the absorbable yin Vital-Qi greater than or equal to 1?"* If you receive a YES, then continue to ask by increasing the figure by 1 number at a time. For example: *"...greater than or equal to 2?"* or *"...greater than or equal to 3?"* until you receive a NO. If you receive a NO while asking *"... greater than or equal to 11?"*, the intensity of the absorbable yin Vital-Qi will be 10 or above. You do not need to do an extra measurement for the value of the absorbable yang Vital-Qi since this will be at least as high or higher than the value for the absorbable yin Vital-Qi.

You can also determine the individual need for absorbable yin Vital-Qi with the tensor or pendulum. The following measuring method is usually adequate for this purpose.

Determining the Individual Need for Absorbable Yin Vital-Qi

The question is: *"Is ... 's (name of the person) individual need for absorbable yin Vital-Qi 9 or higher?"* Increase the numerical value by 0.5 until you receive a NO. Now you have determined the value. The individual requirement is usually between 10 and 12.

In *Correct and Vitalize Your House or Apartment with Feng Shui!* on page 121 ff, we explain how to provide your house or apartment with adequate Vital-Qi in a simple manner.

What is Perm-Qi?

Perm-Qi is an energy that is positive for human beings. It is a certain type of Qi and important for the smooth functioning of the body.

Perm-Qi

Perm-Qi is a type of Qi that is important for the smooth functioning of the body. It is absorbed through our aura, our respiration, and our food. Perm-Qi keeps us physically and mentally fit. We absorb both yang Perm-Qi and yin Perm-Qi. Dependent upon whether the deficiency tends to be related to yang Perm-Qi or yin Perm-Qi, the following symptoms may occur, among others:

A) Yang Perm-Qi Deficiency:
- Decline in general performance
- Burning and stabbing pain in the limbs
- Itching of eyelids with feeling of dryness in eyes
- Involuntary urge to urinate
- Frequent, abundant urination
- Sleepiness during the day

B) Yin Perm-Qi Deficiency:
- Burning and stabbing pain in the joints
- Itching of eyelids without feeling of dryness in eyes
- Fire sparks in front of eyes
- Sleepiness during the day
- Night sweat and reduced hearing can also have a yin Perm-Qi deficiency as contributing factors

Absorbable Perm-Qi

As described under Vital-Qi, there are also two portions to Perm-Qi: the Perm-Qi that human beings can absorb and the type that cannot be absorbed by human beings. Perm-Qi can also always be found as yang Perm-Qi and yin Perm-Qi. Since the values for absorbable yin Perm-Qi are generally lower than the values for absorbable yang Perm-Qi, it is advisable—as already described under Vital-Qi—to only determine the value for absorbable yin Perm-Qi. Both forms of Perm-Qi are measured on a scale from 0 to 100. When we state values for Perm-Qi in the following text, we mean the values for absorbable Perm-Qi. The intensity of Perm-Qi in closed rooms is generally no more than 9 to 12 on this scale. A healthy person actually requires Perm-Qi with a value of 7, but ill or older people need Perm-Qi with a value of 9. Without any special measures, a person can absorb a maximum Perm-Qi value of 12. This value can be increased to 15 through Taijiquan, for example.

Measure Absorbable Yin Perm-Qi with the Tensor or Pendulum!

You have already read how you can measure the absorbable yin Vital-Qi with the tensor or pendulum. Take a similar approach for determining the absorbable yin Perm-Qi.

Measuring the Intensity of Absorbable Yin Perm-Qi

Ask: *"Is the intensity of the absorbable yin Perm-Qi greater than or equal to 2?"* If you receive a YES, then continue to ask by increasing the figure 1 number at a time. For example: *"...greater than or equal to 3?"* or *"...greater than or equal to 4?"* until you receive a NO. If you receive a NO while asking *"...greater than or equal to 11?"*, the intensity of the absorbable yin Perm-Qi will be 10 or just above it. The value of the yang Perm-Qi will be at least as high or higher. You can also determine the individual requirement of absorbable yin Perm-Qi with the tensor or pendulum. The following method is usually adequate for this purpose.

Determining the Individual Need for Absorbable Yin Perm-Qi

The question is: *"Is the individual need for absorbable yin Perm-Qi for ... (name of person) 7 or higher?"* Increase the figure 1 number at a time until you receive a NO. Now you have determined the value. The individual requirement is usually between 7 and 11.

In *Correct and Vitalize Your House or Apartment with Feng Shui!* on page 121 ff, we explain how you can supply your house or apartment with adequate Perm-Qi in a simple manner.

Perm-Qi In the House

There is an adequate amount of Perm-Qi in the **open countryside**. It moves with the air. We can find especially large amounts of Perm-Qi in the vicinity of moving water, such as rivers or the ocean. **Airing the house well** will allow as much Perm-Qi as possible to enter it. This is especially important since only about half of the Perm-Qi will even enter the house. A long time ago, the Chinese already recognized that Perm-Qi not only enters the house with the air, but also discovered that Perm-Qi flows into the opened house door through lens-shaped interfaces. This additional Perm-Qi then moves around the house in two different ways. One portion mixes with the Perm-Qi that has entered the house with the air from the outside. Another portion moves through the house, as described below, on the carrier that it has brought with it from the 4th dimension. The question about absorbable Perm-Qi or absorbable yin Perm-Qi includes this additional Perm-Qi.

What Can Impede Additional Perm-Qi from Entering Your House

The Chinese have always made sure that this additional Perm-Qi actually reaches the inside of the house. They recognized that a mirror installed at a very short distance directly across from the front door does not let any additional Perm-Qi into the house. A wall corner that is located across from the front door also prevents the entry of additional Perm-Qi. In this case, we recommend the placement of a Feng Shui Power Disc 99 in the house.

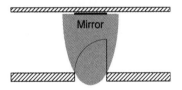

Mirror directly across from the front door.

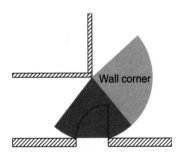

Wall corner directly across from a front door.

How Does the Additional Perm-Qi Move in the House?

The Perm-Qi that additionally comes into the house through open doors, moves in a straight line on its carrier and has the tendency to turn **toward the right** when there are obstacles. This means: if it meets an obstacle and has the possibility of moving to the left or the right, about one-third will turn to the left and two-thirds will turn to the right on its carrier.

On its path through the house, the additional Perm-Qi changes in part from its previous carrier to the **air** and thereby increases the existing air Perm-Qi. There is so much additional Perm-Qi on the carrier that the change to the air can take place over many hours. The longer the path through the house is, the more that air Perm-Qi can be additionally created, which then distributes itself throughout the entire house. This directional behavior can be used in a specific manner by determining the path of the Perm-Qi in the house or apartment through appropriate **placement of the furniture**.

Apart from furniture, **paravents** also have a particularly directing effect on additional Perm-Qi. As much as possible, paravents should be placed in such a way so that the edges do not point directly into the flow of the additional Perm-Qi. **Daylight** and **artificial illumination** also attract additional Perm-Qi. When you want the additional Perm-Qi to flow into certain rooms, be sure that they are well-illuminated.

Within this context, we would like to especially emphasize that **fans are not suitable for directing the additional Perm-Qi**. Instead, fans with fan-like struts of wood reduce the Perm-Qi in a room. This makes them unsuitable for bedrooms in particular.

Additional Perm-Qi Does Not Pass Over Stairs

The additional Perm-Qi on its carrier does not pass over stairs, neither in an upward nor a downward direction. Stairs can even have a negative impact on the flow of the additional Perm-Qi in the house. If there is a staircase leading **upward** directly behind the front door, the additional Perm-Qi on its carrier gets "stuck" on the stairs. As a result, it cannot move to an adequate extent through the rest of the rooms. A staircase that leads **downward** results in the additional Perm-Qi only moving to the uppermost step of the stairs and having difficulty in reaching the rest of the rooms. **Staggered levels** in the house are also a problem for the movement of additional Perm-Qi. Here as well, we recommend the placement of a Feng Shui Power Disc 99 in the house.

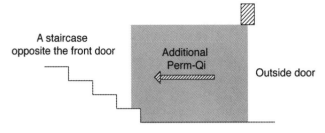

The additional Perm-Qi already "gets stuck" at the first step.

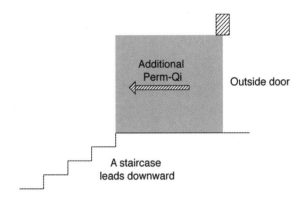

Steps that lead downward are not suited for moving additional Perm-Qi in a downward direction (for example, to the cellar).

Loss of Perm-Qi Because of Long, Straight Passageways in the House

The additional Perm-Qi normally tends to move slowly (about 1/2 meter or yard a second) on its carrier through a story of a house. If there are long, straight passageways, its speed will increase. If a critical speed is exceeded in the process, it disappears into a higher dimension. We therefore recommend (also because of other feng shui reasons) that you slow down the speed of the additional Perm-

Qi in such passageways by using suitable measures. There are a number of possibilities for doing this that also have a favorable effect on the movement of the Perm-Qi.

Placing Pieces of Furniture or Plants in Straight Passageways

The placement of pieces of furniture or plants on the right side (seen from the flow direction of the additional Perm-Qi) leads to a relative slowing of the speed.

Plants
or furniture

Additional
Perm-Qi

The placement of plants or furniture in straight passageways on the right side (in the flow direction of the additional Perm-Qi).

Illumination in Straight Passageways

The placement of illumination on the right side leads to a slowing down of the flow of additional Perm-Qi. Moreover, it is attracted in an upward direction from light source to light source. This also leads to a slowing down of the overall flow. For this purpose, the illumination should be installed in the upper half of the wall or to the right on the ceiling.

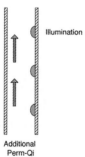

Illumination

Additional
Perm-Qi

Illumination in straight passageways on the right side (in the flow direction of the additional Perm-Qi).

Additional Perm-Qi Escapes through the Window

The additional Perm-Qi on its carrier has the tendency of moving toward the light. After a certain stretch of the house, it therefore generally moves to a window and disappears there at an interface in the window into a higher dimension. It therefore "leaves" the house. This is particularly the case when the window is located directly across from the front door.

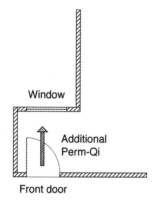

Additional Perm-Qi "disappears" through the window into a higher dimension. This is particularly the case for a window opposite a front door.

Wind Chimes Prevent Additional Perm-Qi from Escaping through the Window

Wind chimes for this purpose are made of metal or glass pipes of various lengths. When wind chimes are hung in front of a window, they practically form a curtain of energy that prevents the additional Perm-Qi from escaping into a higher dimension. They do not have to be struck for this purpose, but they must be able to sound. If possible, the wind chimes in a room should be hung at a distance of about 40 centimeters from the window. In doing so, they should be placed in the upper third of the window and at about the center of the window width.

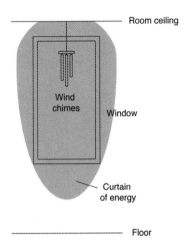

Wind chimes in front of the window can prevent the additional Perm-Qi from escaping. It has the effect of a curtain of energy.

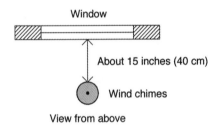

It is best to hang wind chimes at a distance of about 15 inches (40 cm) from the window.

Wind chimes should never have black pipes. Also avoid yellow wind chimes, at least in front of a window. On the other hand, gold or brass-colored wind chimes are not considered yellow and are therefore beneficial.

Wind chimes should never be hung behind the balcony door or the front door since this hinders the additional Perm-Qi from entering the house.

Additional Perm-Qi Also Disappears through the Toilet

Additional Perm-Qi disappears into a higher dimension through the **drain pipe** of the toilet. This also applies to a much lesser extent to other drain pipes. A toilet should not be located across from the front door or to the right adjacent to it. Toilet lids and doors to the toilet should be kept closed. This reduces the loss of additional Perm-Qi. In addition, you should place a Feng Shui Power Disc 99 in the house.

Daylight and Perm-Qi

Daylight in the interior rooms plays an important role. It can even contribute to an increase of the air Perm-Qi. However, light that is too bright should be avoided.

Artificial Illumination and Perm-Qi

Within this context, the function of daylight can also be largely taken over by artificial illumination. All customary sources of artificial light are suitable for this purpose. However, please observe our comments on electrical illumination in the section on *Feng Shui and Electrosmog* on page 154 ff.

Increasing the Perm-Qi through Sounded Wind Chimes

Sounded wind chimes increase the absorbable Perm-Qi in a room for many hours. The Perm-Qi created by the sound is a further possibility of getting more Perm-Qi into a room, along with additional Perm-Qi and Perm-Qi through light. This Perm-Qi also increases the existing Perm-Qi in the room. According to its construction type and size, the wind chimes should be sounded once or more frequently every day. We particularly recommend vigorously sounding the wind chimes before you go to sleep at night. Here as well, be sure that the wind chimes never have black pipes.

Increasing the Perm-Qi in the Entire House through One Single Feng Shui Remedy

In the next chapter, we describe how you can distinctly increase the Perm-Qi in the entire house through the Feng Shui Power Disc 99 or the so-called Tachyonized Silica Discs in a special arrangement.

Chapter 5

Correct and Vitalize Your House or Apartment with Feng Shui!

In this book, we wanted to present three basic possibilities for protecting yourself against both familiar and additional negative influences that have not yet been described, as well as intensifying positive energies.

The first and best possibility consists of practically "dissolving" the disruptive subtle and non-material structures of the 3rd dimension in an entire house completely and strengthening the inner and outer aura structure of the house. (The aura structure of the house is described in Chapter 7 on page 165 ff) Then you will be effectively protected against Geo-Sha, Trans-Sha through metals, Trans-Sha, and Per-Sha and the positive energies in the house will be increased. In addition, this will have a good effect on a large number of another feng shui problems in the house. In order to achieve this, you can use the **Feng Shui Power Disc 99** that we will introduce in this chapter.

The second best possibility is to use the so-called **Tachyonized Silica Discs.** When arranged properly, negative energies (Geo-Sha, Trans-Sha through metals, Trans-Sha, and Per-Sha) in the entire house will also be reduced and positive energies increased. You can also dissolve disruptive subtle and non-material structures of the 3rd dimension in the house with the Tachyonized Silica Discs. However, the effect on the inner and outer aura structure of the house is not as pronounced; as a result, the effect on many other feng shui problems in the house is not adequate.

The third possibility consists of just reducing the negative energies in a limited area without considerably increasing the positive energies at the same time. Disruptive subtle and non-material structures of the 3rd dimension in the house will also not be dissolved as a result of this measure. In this context, we will discuss *XEPS plates, cellular glass slabs of a suitable quality, and cork tiles of a suitable quality.*

New Structures Come from the 4th and 5th Dimension

The disruptive structures in the house (10-Meter System, 250-Meter System, etc.) are connected to the existence of the 0.67-Centimeter System. If the 0.67-Centimeter System is "dissolved," both of the 0.95-Centimeter Systems, as well as the larger disruptive structures, will dissolve. In order to dissolve the 0.67-Centimeter System, the following possibilities are available: You can replace the 0.67-Centimeter System with a suitable conductive system of the 4th and 5th dimension, in which the 0.67-Centimeter System is accelerated into the 2nd dimension. Then the larger disruptive cube systems in the house will disappear as well. These include:

- The 10-Meter System
- The 250-Meter System
- The 170-Meter System
- The Hartmann System
- Moon stripes
- The Curry System
- The 400-Meter System complex (only with the Feng Shui Power Disc 99)

Consequently, no undesired energies with their carriers—such as Geo-Sha, Trans-Sha, and Per-Sha from the 5th or 4th dimension—can be accelerated into our dimension.

The following structures and the interfaces that they have within them are either changed or prevented from developing, which means that there will virtually be no more harmful structures and harmful energies

- Structures above watercourses
- Structures above fault zones

The appropriate conductive systems of the 4th and 5th dimension can be accelerated into the 3rd dimension by means of the feng shui remedies. This occurs through the suitable interfaces, which become effective accordingly. The conductive system of the 4th dimension that is accelerated into the 3rd dimension consists of the flowing walls in cube forms of various sizes. The conductive system of the 5th dimension that is accelerated into the 3rd dimension consists of pipes of various sizes and directions in space.

The conductive systems of the 4th and 5th dimension that are accelerated into the 3rd dimension spread out in the house. When the Feng Shui Power Disc 99 is used, this expansion moves beyond the aura structure of the house and also effects the property around it. When the Tachyonized Silica Discs are used in the appropriate arrangement, the expansion is limited to the aura structure of the house.

The new structures in the house contain interfaces through which energies that are positive for us—such as Vital-Qi, Perm-Qi, and Shen—are accelerated from the 5th dimension into our dimension. The energies also bring their carriers along from the 5th dimension into our 3rd dimension. These carriers provide a continuing good supply of positive energies for the house.

The Feng Shui Power Disc 99

The Feng Shui Power Disc 99 provides adequate protection against Geo-Sha, Trans-Sha, Trans-Sha through metals, and the various types of Per-Sha in the house. The basis for this effect is, as already described above, the dissolution or the replacement of the 0.67-Centimeter System through a conductive system of the 4th dimension in combination with a conductive system of the 5th dimension. The larger cube systems (for example, the 10-Meter, 250-Meter, 170-Meter, Hartmann, and Curry System and the 400-Meter System complex) are also dissolved or replaced in the process.

The Feng Shui Power Disc 99 will bring subtle positive energies into the house, including Vital-Qi, Perm-Qi, and Shen. The Feng Shui Power Disc 99 also leads to a greater equilibrium of the Five Elements (see *Wu Xing: The Five Laws of Change* on page 166 ff). In addition, with the Feng Shui Power Disc 99 you can distinctly improve or resolve a majority of the feng shui problems in your house. There is an overview of important additional effects at the end of this chapter. (For supply sources, see "Information and Advice" in the appendix.)

The Placement of the Feng Shui Power Disc 99

The Feng Shui Power Disc 99 is simply hung on the wall in the house. A precise description with additional details on placement is included with the Feng Shui Power Disc 99. One single Feng Shui Power Disc 99 is also adequate for larger houses and plots of land. We can assume that one Feng Shui Power Disc 99 can be used for the above purposes for a period of about 50 years. However, its materials must remain intact—it should not be broken or damaged in any way.

A Good Night's Sleep Because of the Feng Shui Power Disc

After a feng shui consultation, a Feng Shui Power Disc was hung up in a duplex house. A few days later, the neighbor, who lived in the adjoining duplex and knew nothing of the feng shui consultation, reported that he had been able to sleep through the night for the past few days. Now he no longer woke up around 2 a.m. and had to watch television for a while. He had no explanation for this change in his sleeping habits since his sleep disorder had been chronic for years.

Tachyonized Silica Discs

Some years ago, Japanese scientists succeeded in using an electrical vacuum to change various materials in their submolecular structure. Such a process lasts about 3 weeks. The American David Wagner found to way to translate this new technology into practical terms, which he named "tachyonization."

The tachyonized products also include the so-called tachyonized silica disc. These discs has a diameter of 4 inches (10 cm), which are currently provided with a straightened edge of up to 12/8 inches (4 cm) in one or two places. The silica discs have lettering on one side. They are also used for therapeutic purposes (see *Information and Advice* on page 243).

Two Silica Discs in a Special Arrangement

You will require two silica discs to protect your house against Geo-Sha, Trans-Sha, and Trans-Sha through metals, as well as for increasing Vital-Qi and Perm-Qi. Be sure to observe the special arrangement of the discs: The two silica discs are installed with one above the other in a horizontal direction. There should be an air layer of 2/8 inches (min. 1/2 in., max. 5/16 in.) or 6 mm (min. 3 mm, max. 8 mm) between the two silica discs. Without this air layer, they will not have an adequate effect. The upper silica disc should have its lettering pointing in an upward direction, and the lower silica disc should have its lettering pointing downward. It is necessary to place the **lower** silica disc (with the lettered side pointing downward) in an empty, clear, colorless CD case. The distance between the two silica discs will now be just less than 5/16 inches (just under 8 mm). Please be sure that you **definitely do not** place the upper silica disc in an empty CD case as well since the distance between the two silica discs would then be too great.

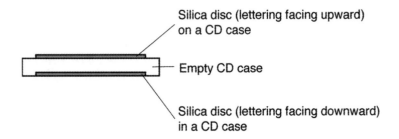

Two silica discs in and on a CD case in a special arrangement

Distance to the room wall: Align the CD case so that it is parallel to the room walls that match the orientation of the house. The distance between the CD case and the room wall should be at least 4 inches (10 cm) and at most 21 inches (55 cm).

Distance to the room ceiling and floor: The distance to the room ceiling should be at least 14 inches (35 inches) and at least 16 inches (40 cm) to the floor. When both silica discs are placed in a room in which you frequently spend time, it is advantageous to place the two silica discs above the level of the head. You can, for example, place them on a high closest or other piece of furniture that is tall enough.

We recommend that you replace the silica discs with new ones for the feng shui remedies described here after about 8 years or at least check the effectiveness of the feng shui remedies.

There are two placement possibilities:
A) Place the discs in the house outside of the side walls of the appropriate direction-dependent cube system.
B) Place the discs in the house within the side wall of the appropriate direction-dependent cube system (for example: the 10-Meter, 250-Meter, Hartmann, and 170-Meter System, as well as the 400-Meter System complex).

A) Placement of the silica discs outside of the side wall of the appropriate direction-dependent cube system

In one-family houses, it is best to place both silica discs on the first floor. A placement in about the middle of the floor place is best, but not absolutely necessary. In addition to the floor on which they are placed, both of the discs have an impact on at least 4 stories above and at least 2 stories below. For larger houses, it may be beneficial to place them in the second floor. The radius of the effect is about 115 feet (35 m).

Such a placement provides adequate protection against Geo-Sha, Trans-Sha, and Trans-Sha through metals. The Vital-Qi and Perm-Qi will also be distinctly increased. However, the larger direction-dependent structures in the house will not be dissolved. Problems that result because of certain Form School situations (such as sharp corners and edges, etc.) will not be improved. The protection against Per-Sha 61 above fault zones, Per-Sha 36 in the case of clock radios with a red digital display, as well as Per-Sha caused by satellite dishes is partially inadequate.

For houses that do not have a parallelepiped shape or have a slanting roof, the generally preferred location for the disc is outside the appropriate wall in the side wall of the appropriate cube system. This situation will be described in the next section.

B) Placement of the silica disc in the side wall of the appropriate direction-dependent cube system

Use the same arrangement of the two silica discs and the CD case, as described above. The distance to the wall, etc., should also be as described above. This type of placement is suitable for the following systems, among others: The 10-Meter, 250-Meter, Hartmann, and 170-Meter System, as well as the 400-Meter System complex. It is possible to place the disc in either the main wall or the secondary wall of the 400-Meter System complex. When placed in such a manner, the protection is also adequate for floors with slanted roofs and houses that are not parallelepiped-shaped. As described under placement A), the two silica discs have an effect on at least 4 stories above the floor upon which they have been place and at least 2 stories below. In larger houses, a placement on the second floor can also be advantageous. For this placement, the radius of the effect is about 130 feet (40 m).

This placement results in an adequate protection against Geo-Sha, Trans-Sha, and Trans-Sha through metals, as well as an even more intense increase in Vital-Qi and Perm-Qi. A variety of larger direction-dependent structures in the house are dissolved (for example: the 10-Meter, 250-Meter, Hartmann, and 170-Meter System; however, this is inadequate for the 400-Meter System complex). Problems that result on the basis of certain Form School situations (such as sharp corners and edges, etc.) are also not improved. The protection against Per-Sha 36 in the case of clock radios with red digital displays is partially inadequate.

However, we should remember that the direction-dependent structures that are suitable for the placement of silica discs can also be shifted through external influences (for example, movable metals like parked cars). The way in which the Tachyonized Silica Discs expand their effect in the house is similar to that described under the section on the Feng Shui Power Disc 99.

A Student Wakes Up with a Morning Headache on a Regular Basis

A student complained at a party for doctoral candidates that he frequently already had a headache when he woke up in the morning. A feng shui consultant, who also had been invited to the party, offered to examine his studio apartment the following week. When walking through the apartment, she noticed that the metal portion of the electrical appliances in the kitchen next to the bedroom caused Trans-Sha through metals to be focused with a great intensity upon the head end of the bed because of the thin room wall. In this case, the remedy was two Tachyonized Silica Discs that were placed in a special arrangement in the apartment. The headaches disappeared by the next morning. Moreover, about 1 week after the placement of the silica discs, the student reported that he also felt fresher during the day and could work in a more concentrate manner.

Invisible Structures Resembling
a Faraday Cage

There are materials that do not have an impact on the entire house but partially protect us like a "Faraday Cage," even if the mode of action is completely different. In the effective area of these materials (protective structure) lens and spirals are so changed in their function that almost no more Geo-Sha and almost no more Trans-Sha is created in our dimension in this area. This only applies partially to Per-Sha (see under the individual materials). The Sha is not conducted away and is also not shielded or filtered by the material; instead, it is not in the first place. Within this protective structure, no acceleration of Sha into our dimension takes place. However, the direction-dependent structures remain in place. Furthermore, we must remember that Qi is generally not increased to an adequate degree in this case.

The following materials are particularly suited for creating such protective structures: **XEPS plates, cork tiles of a suitable quality,** and **cellular glass slabs of a suitable quality.** Since every material is made of a somewhat different structure and keeps for a different length of time, it is necessary to discuss the individual materials separately.

XEPS Plates

XEPS plates (extruded polystyrene hard-foam plates) consist of plastic. They are made of closed-cell polystyrene foam that has been rolled (extruded) under pressure. XEPS plates have a smooth surface and are primarily used for the heat insulation of buildings. They have an extremely low ability to conduct heat, a considerable resistance to pressure, as well as being resistant to rot and the change between frost and dew. They can be used for both the heat insulation of flat roofs and the perimeter insulation of floors in the ground-floor area.

In the USA, XEPS plates are offered for sale in the quality required for the feng shui purposes described here by DOW Chemical. In the USA and Canada, the standard size of the plates is 24 x 96 inches (125 x 60 cm in Europe). The plates can be purchased in specialized building material stores starting at a thickness of 1 inch (in Europe, starting at 2 cm). The following plates are suitable for this purpose: Styrofoam High Load 40, Styrofoam High Load 60, and Styrofoam High Load 100. The following suitable plates can be ordered in Germany: Fina X by Isofoam, Styrodur by BASF, and Jackodur by Gefinex. The product Roofmate made by the Dow Chemical Company is also suitable. However, this product is not identical with the Roofmate product in the USA.

Protective Structure through Horizontally Laid XEPS Plates

Horizontally laid XEPS plates create the desired protective structure. They build up this structure in both a downward and an upward direction. We therefore can find almost no Geo-Sha and Trans-Sha in the side walls of the corresponding cube systems. In addition, metals located placed in the side walls bring almost no additional Trans-Sha into the room. This means that the XEPS plates give adequate protection both above, as well as below, the plate. Regarding the effect of Per-Sha, please see the chart at the end of this chapter. We find an minor increase of Perm-Qi directly above the XEPS plates, up to a height of about 3 feet (1 m), in as far as the XEPS plates are not located in the side wall of the 10-Meter or 250-Meter System.

When there are square plates, the length of the structure in the upward direction consists of more than 3.6 times that of the diagonal lines, measured from the plate. If several plates are placed in a row, the diagonal line of the entire surface is counted. A **minimum surface** of about 7.5 **square feet (0.75 square m)** is required for building the structure in an upward direction. However, in order to build the structure completely down to the ground, a **minimum surface** of 10.5 **square feet (1 square m)** is necessary.

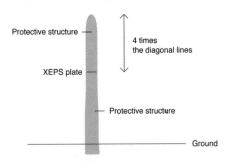

Invisible protective structures through horizontally laid XEPS plates: In an upward direction, the structure consists of 3.6 times the diagonal lines; it reaches the ground in a downward direction.

Length of the Effect for the XEPS Plates

The effect of the XEPS plates for the above-described feng shui purposes is limited in terms of time: In relation to Geo-Sha, Trans-Sha, and Trans-Sha through metals, this is about 9 years after they have been completed.

Using XEPS Plates in the Home

One example is to use the XEPS plates extensively as heat insulation in the foundation plate of the house or in the cellar. They can also be used as footfall insulation in false ceilings. It is also possible to just lay them under the bed or under metals, for example.

When installing them, be aware that XEPS plates only develop their effect, which means building the appropriate structure, when they are laid in a strictly horizontal manner. In old buildings with somewhat slanted floors, it may be necessary to use a spirit level.

The protective structure continues upward,
up to four times the diagonal lines of the XEPS plate
or the XEPS plates located next to each other

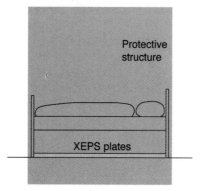

The protective structure continues in a downward direction

A bed is underlaid with the XEPS plates.

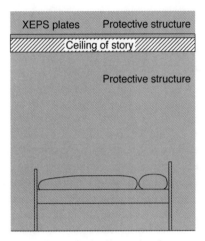

The floor in the story above the bedroom has been covered with XEPS plates.

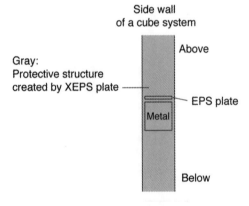

An XEPS plate can be laid either above or below the metal.

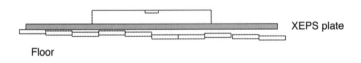

When floors are slanted or uneven, the horizontal laying of XEPS plates must be checked with a spirit level.

XEPS Plates: Good for Health and Well-Being

A 45-year-old car mechanic had already stopped working several years before due to health reasons. He suffered from years of jaw pain and depression and did not feel capable of working, even though he very much enjoyed his work. A feng shui inspection at his home revealed, among other things, a series of problems caused by Geo-Sha and Trans-Sha. Since he had planned to lay new wooden floors, as well as heat insulation, in the ground floor of his house, this opportunity was used to install XEPS plates beneath the entire living room. Since the largest portion of the bedroom was situated above the living room, the bedroom was also protected by the structure above the XEPS plates. In the following months, the master mechanic reported on the improvements:

His sleep had improved; the jaw complaints subsided and his general state of health, as well as his mood, gradually improved. His small son also slept more peacefully and the children particularly liked to play on the floor of the living room, which they had previously tended to avoid. The entire family life shifted from the kitchen into the living room.

XEPS Plates Should Not Be Employed Vertically

At times, we also find XEPS plates as heat-insulation material for house walls. If the XEPS plates point directly in one of the main directions (north, east, south, or west), there is the possibility that inauspicious energies can get into the house. Check the directions to be avoided with a tensor or pendulum. You will usually determine a deviation of between 2.5 and 5 degrees to the west when looking to the geographic direction of north. In this manner, the XEPS plates are effective for up to about 11 years, meaning that they stop being effective about 11 years after the house has been built. If you have problems with vertically installed XEPS plates in your house, you can use a Feng Shui Power Disc 99 for protection.

Cellular Glass Slabs of a Suitable Quality

The primary material for the manufacture of cellular glass is sand. Special additives allow a high-grade type of glass to be created in the first stage of production. This product is subsequently extruded, crushed, and then ground into a glass powder. Combined with carbon, the glass powder is heated in an oven at about 1000 degrees Celsius. In the process, the carbon oxidizes and gas bubbles are formed during the foaming process. Afterward, the material is slowly cooled in an expanding oven.

Cellular glass is waterproof, steamproof, non-combustible, will not rot, and is resistant to pressure, acid, and pests.

Cellular glass slabs of a suitable quality offer adequate protection against Geo-Sha, Trans-Sha, and Trans-Sha through metals. (With regard to Per-Sha, please see the chart at the end of the chapter.) The following products are suitable for the feng shui purposes described here: Foamglas HLB 1400 or HLB 1600 and Foamglas Board HLB 1400 or 1600 by the Pittsburgh Corning Company in a thickness of 2 inches. Standard sizes are 24 x 18 inches, 12 x 18 inches, and 24 x 48 inches. In Europe, use the Foamglas F or Foamglass Floorboard F by Pittsburgh Corning in a thickness of 5 centimeters.

Protective Structure through Horizontally Laid Cellular Glass Slabs of a Suitable Quality

In terms of building an invisible structure, the horizontally laid cellular glass slabs behave in the same way as the XEPS plates. The only difference is that the upward height of the structure consists of at least 3.3 times that of the diagonal line in square slabs. The minimum area for the complete formation of the structure, in both an upward and downward direction to the ground, consists of 2.5 square feet (0.25 square m).

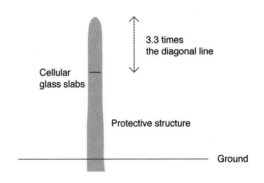

Protective structure through horizontally laid cellular glass slabs.

Length of the Effect

The length of the effect of cellular glass slabs is 60 years and longer.

Use of Cellular Glass Slabs

Cellular glass slabs can be laid horizontally in the following manner according to the feng shui approach:

a) Under foundation plates of houses and high-rise buildings
b) Above the floor plate beneath cement floors
c) In agriculture; for example, in the foundation plates of barns

Their good resistance to wear makes it particularly feasible to use these in places where it is not possible to exchange materials. For houses that have a height of about 60 feet (20 m), cellular glass can also be used for shielding from above by installing it in flat roofs. For lower houses, a covering from above is not recommended from the perspective of feng shui. Use in a roof overhang is also inadvisable from the perspective of feng shui.

When the roof overhangs of a house project beyond the foundation plate, the surface outside the foundation plate beneath the roof overhangs should also be laid out with cellular glass, in as far as you do not use the Feng Shui Power Disc 99. This is particularly important when the eaves and gutters are made of metal or other types of metals are attached to the house. Balconies should also be underlaid with cellular glass, especially when they have railings made of metal.

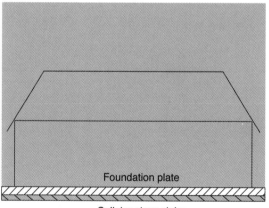

Foundation plate

Cellular glass slabs

Cellular glass slabs must be laid beneath the house in such a way that all walls, roof overhangs, and balconies are included in the protective structure.

135

A Balcony Is "Corrected"

A woman had been suffering from chronic pain for years. Her bed was taken out of the side wall of the 10-Meter System. However, Trans-Sha with a strong intensity continued to come from the heavy metal railing of the balcony, reaching even the new sleeping place. The problem was solved by gluing cellular glass slabs directly under the balcony from below. This created the desired protection for the bedroom.

Cork Tiles of a Suitable Quality

Cork tiles of a suitable quality have been used for many years now to successfully correct sleeping environments. The primary material for cork tiles is the bark of the cork oak (Quercus suber lin.). Unfortunately, the cork qualities and grades of thickness of the tiles offered by the trade are often unsuitable. Either they contain too much adhesive or inappropriate filler material like wood waste. In addition, the plates are unsuitable when a cork granulate of a peeling is used that does not build up enough of a structure with adequate mass (for example, the first peeling). Tiles with a thickness of 5/16 to 9/16 inches (8 to 15 mm) are suitable; thicker tiles can also be used. The cork tiles have a standard size of about 24 x 36 inches (in Europe, 61 x 91.5 cm), but cork parquet with a thickness of 5/16 to 6/16 inches (8 to 10 mm) is also suitable. Cork tiles or cork parquet of a suitable quality is only available through select supply addresses (see appendix under "Information and Advice"). They also provide adequate protection against Geo-Sha, Trans-Sha, and Trans-Sha through metals. In terms of the effect on Per-Sha, please see the chart at the end of this chapter. We find an minor increase of Perm-Qi directly above the cork tiles, up to a height of about 3 feet (1 m), in as far as the cork tiles are not located in the side wall of the 10-Meter or 250-Meter System.

Protective Structure through Horizontally Laid Cork Tiles of a Suitable Quality

In contrast to XEPS plates and cellular glass slabs, which should only be laid in a horizontal direction, cork tiles can be applied successfully for correcting the sleeping environment in both the horizontal and the vertical directions.

Horizontally laid cork tiles of a suitable quality in the customary format (24 x 36 inches or 61 x 91.5 cm) build a protective structure above and below the cork tiles. However, this structure is formed somewhat differently than that of the XEPS plates and the cellular glass slabs. For square cork tiles, the upward length of the structure consists of more than twice the diagonal line at the center (above about 25% of the overall surface) measured from the tile itself. In addition to this, the length of the structure consists of at least just less than the diagonal measurement, whereby a total of about 20% of the surface portion at the edge of the cork tile is left out. The minimum surface for completely building the structure in an upward direction is 2.5 square feet (0.25 m). The minimum surface for building a structure down to the ground is even less than 2.5 square feet (0.25 square m).

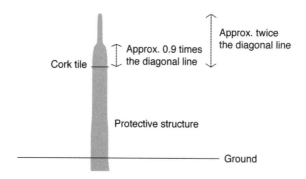

Protective structure through horizontally laid cork tiles that are not square.

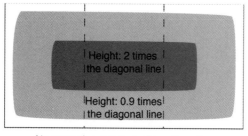

No protective structure above the edge

Protective structure through horizontally laid cork tiles that are not square (top view).

Special Characteristics for Cork Parquet or for Square Cork Tiles

Cork parquet of a suitable quality consists of individual square tiles. We find a uniform protective structure with a height of 1.9 times the diagonal line above square cork tiles of a suitable quality.

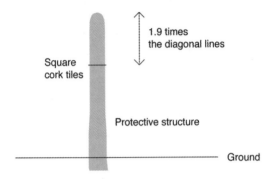

Protective structure through horizontally laid square cork tiles.

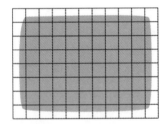

Protective structure through horizontally laid square cork tiles (top view).

Length of Effect for Horizontal Installation

Cork tiles have a long service life in relation to Geo-Sha, Trans-Sha and Per-Sha. The length of this service life can be increased through appropriate care. This includes airing it two or three times a year on dry, sunny days. The tiles should be protected from moisture. Be sure that the cork tiles, if possible, are not laid directly under the mattress. If these points are observed, their durability consists of 40 years and longer.

Horizontal Application of Suitable Cork Tiles

Cork tiles can basically be used like the XEPS plates. However, keep in mind that the upward height of the structure is considerably less and that there is an unprotected zone at the edges of the laid surfaces. So a larger surface is required for adequate upward protection.

Cork tiles are frequently laid under the **bed** (on the floor). Since the standard size is 24 x 36 inches (61 x 91.5 cm), at least 3 tiles are required in order to protect a larger sleeping surface. Take into consideration that there is an unprotected zone above the edge of the cork tiles. Be absolutely sure that the individual cork tiles are right up against each other. You can use sturdy adhesive tape to hold them in place. Should only 3 tiles be laid, ensure that the head and other strained body parts are adequately protected.

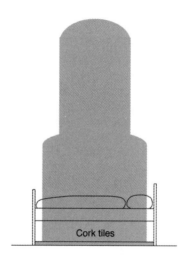

Protective structure through horizontally laid cork tiles when bed is completely underlaid (side view).

It is also good to underlay **metal furnishing objects**. However, when doing so you should ensure that these interior decorating objects are located as completely as possible within the structure built by the cork tile. In addition, cork tiles can be laid above metal objects when this is feasible. Laying cork tiles under carpeting is also a possibility. However, when they are laid out without being attached, the cork tiles do not provide the desired durability so that using cork parquet tends to be a better approach.

Horizontal Application of Suitable Cork Parquet

When laying a large area, we recommend that you use cork parquet since this is quite durable. When doing so, be sure that the cork parquet has a minimum thickness of 5/16 inches (8 mm). The cork parquet that is usually offered in building-supply stores is usually too thin and is also unsuitable in terms of its quality for improving the sleeping environment (see *Information and Advice* on page 243). Technical skill is required to lay cork parquet and this work should be left up to a specialist if you have any doubts about your ability to do it. The parquet should be glued to a smooth background and then sealed or treated with wax.

Cork Parquet Instead of an Operation

A feng shui consultant, who works together with a physician, reported the following: "The 45-year-old Ms. S. suffered from acute rheumatism. Her knees were affected in particular. Already she had consulted all of the known doctors and healing practitioners in the immediate and more distant surroundings, but the symptoms increasingly worsened. She even had difficulty in walking on crutches. Although she had previously enjoyed going window-shopping, she now stayed at home as much as possible, often even in bed. When I did a feng shui examination of the house, she had just received the news that her right knee was to be replaced by an endoprosthesis. In addition, her left knee was to be operated on at a later date, after she regained the use of her right leg. She slept with both knees in a side wall of the 10-Meter System. A closet with mirror doors was also located within this side wall so that she was also being affected from the side.

She and her husband decided to lay cork parquet in the room directly beneath the bedroom; in addition, the closet with mirror doors was replaced by a new bedroom closet without a mirror. In this case, simply correcting the sleeping area with a feng shui approach was not adequate. The strain on the patient had to be additionally reduced. Ms. S. chose therapy with the WS Frequency Device. After her knees had been irradiated for a total of nine times with the WS Frequency Device, I ran into Ms. S. in the downtown area. Although she still walked quite slowly, she was almost free of pain. After four more weeks, I met her again in a supermarket and her condition had once again improved."

Protection for the Entire House through Cork Parquet

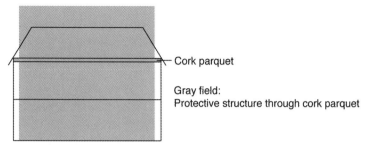

Cork parquet

Gray field:
Protective structure through cork parquet

Correcting a large area by using cork parquet is possible on the uppermost floor. Here: laying it in an attic that has been turned into living space.

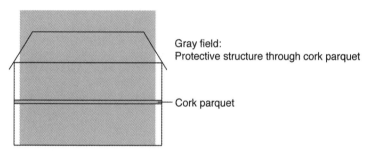

Gray field:
Protective structure through cork parquet

Cork parquet

It is also useful to lay cork parquet in the middle of the house as protection for the entire house.

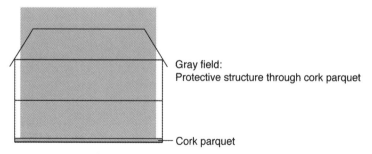

Gray field:
Protective structure through cork parquet

Cork parquet

When you lay cork parquet in the ground floor of a house, the house should not be higher than the protection through the protective structure.

Protective Structure through Vertically Applied Cork Tiles
of a Suitable Quality

Vertically applied cork tiles of a suitable quality also build up a protective structure. However, this is smaller than that of the horizontal application. The structure is only formed to the side of the surfaces. It has a length to each side of approx. 1.2 times the diagonal line of the cork tile, whereby a minimum surface starting at about 10.5 square feet (1 square m) almost achieves the maximum effect of the structure. In the process, the edge of the cork tile has no structure. This unprotected part at each edge consists of about 10% of the height or width of the cork plate.

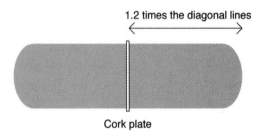

Protective structure through vertically applied cork tiles.

Effect of the Structure through Vertically Applied Suitable
Cork Tiles

The primary effect of this structure is that Trans-Sha is not activated by the metals in the side walls of the 10-Meter or 250-Meter System. The same also applies for metals in the side walls of the 170-Meter and Hartmann System.

Length of the Effect in Vertical Application

The length of the effect is comparable to the length for horizontal application and consists of 40 years or more.

Vertical Application of Suitable Cork Tiles

Cork tiles can also be applied to the side of metals in order to prevent them from activating Trans-Sha. This applies to both visible metals and metals that are not visible, such as those that may present problems in the form of iron girders in staggered levels of a house.

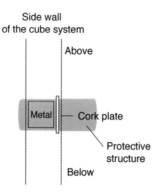

Side wall
of the cube system

Above

Metal — Cork plate

Protective
structure

Below

Cork tiles can also be applied to the side of metals so that no Trans-Sha is activated in the side wall of a cube system.

Steel Girders and Staggered Levels

A couple lived in a row house on a hillside. Among other things, a feng shui examination revealed a considerable negative impact on the matrimonial bed caused by Trans-Sha, which came out of the wall at the head of the bed. The bedroom wall itself was neither in the wall of the 10-Meter nor the 250-Meter System. So the negative impact must originate in the neighboring house. The couple was certain that the neighbors had no large metal objects located within the entire house. When the feng shui consultant persistently asked whether metal objects had been used in the construction of the house, it turned out that massive steel girders had been installed. Because of the hillside location, the neighboring row house had been built in a staggered position so that the steel girders were placed in the bedroom wall exactly above the heads of the couple. The bedroom walls were then sufficiently covered with cork tiles at this place. Combined with therapy, this remedy caused the symptoms to quickly subside.

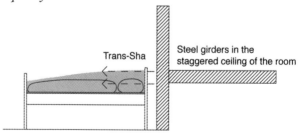

Trans-Sha

Steel girders in the
staggered ceiling of the room

A steel girder brings Trans-Sha to the bed.

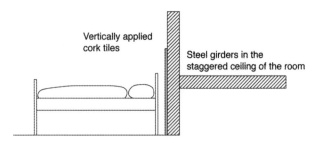

Cork tiles were applied vertically.

Non-Extruded Styrofoam Is Not a Shielding Material

Non-extruded styrofoam (such as Cellofoam) is not a shielding material; however, in individual cases it can impair the effect of the shielding materials described above or, in rare cases, it may even amplify them.

Non-extruded styrofoam should not be used in a horizontal direction when constructing a house. However, it is suitable as heat insulation in house walls (vertical).

A Comparison of Feng Shui Remedies for Correcting and Vitalizing

Now you have become familiar with the various feng shui remedies for correcting and vitalizing. These feng shui remedies can be basically divided into two groups:

1) Feng shui remedies that reduce Sha and increase Qi in the entire house, also dissolving the relevant direction-dependent structures, if necessary.
2) Feng shui remedies that only reduce Sha in a specific area, without essentially increasing the Qi or dissolving the relevant direction-dependent structures.

The first group of feng shui measures includes the placement of a Feng Shui Power Disc 99 in the house, as well as (with a somewhat more limited effect) the appropriate placement of two Tachyonized Silica Discs in the house.

The second group of feng shui remedies includes covering one section of the house or the entire floor space with XEPS plates, cellular glass plates of a suitable quality, or cork plate/cork parquet of a suitable quality. The remedies of the second group are generally more complicated in technical terms and, when it comes to the bottom line, also more cost intensive than the remedies of the first group.

The following chart provides a comparative overview of the feng shui remedies that have been described up to now:

Overview: Comparison of the Feng Shui Remedies

	Feng Shui Power Disc 99	Silica Discs	XEPS Plates	Cellular Glass (Foamglas F)	Cork of a Suitable Quality
Upward Shielding effect	Also adequate for larger houses	At least 4 stories above the floor where the 2 silica discs are placed.	3.6 x the diagonal	3.3 x the diagonal	'Non-square plates: Double structure 0.9 x and 2 x the diagonal. Square plates (cork parquet): 1.9 x diagonal
Downward shielding effect	Also adequate for larger houses	At least 2 stories below the floor where the 2 silica discs are placed.	To the cellar	To the cellar	To the cellar
Sideways shielding effect	To plot boundaries	115 to 130 feet (35 to 40 m)	Structure extends a little to side beyond edge of plate	Structure extends a little to side beyond edge of plate	Structure does not cover entire surface of cork tiles
Minimum surface for adequate effect	1 Feng Shui Power Disc 99	2 normal silica discs and 1 CD case	10.5 square feet (1 sq. m)	2.5 square feet (0.25 sq. m)	2.5 square feet (0.25 sq. m)
Reduction of Geo-Sha and Trans-Sha	100% (99% above watercourses)	99 to 100%	98%	96%	95%
Dissolution of direction-dependent structures	Yes	Only when placed in side wall of appropriate cube system	No	No	No
Increase of Vital-Qi	Clear increase of Vital-Qi	Clear increase of Vital-Qi	None	None	None
Increase of Perm-Qi	Clear increase of Perm-Qi	Clear increase of Perm-Qi	Inadequate	Inadequate	Inadequate
Durability for feng shui purposes	Approx. 50 yrs.	8 yrs.	At least 8 yrs.	60 yrs.	40 yrs.

	Feng Shui Power Disc 99	Silica Discs	XEPS Plates	Cellular Glass (Foamglas F)	Cork of a Suitable Quality
Special characteristics	• Also has good effect on many other feng shui problems in the house	• When placed in the side wall of an appropriate cube system, effect is stronger on roof overhangs	• Strict horizontal installation required	• Only select qualities are adequately effective	• Only select qualities are adequately effective

Here is an extra chart to illustrate the special characteristics that result in the effect on Per-Sha.

Overview: Comparison of Effects on Per-Sha

	Feng Shui Power Disc 99	Silica Discs	XEPS Plates	Cellular Glass (Foamglas F)	Cork of a Suitable Quality
Reduction of Per-Sha 36 (from clock radios with red digital display) (strain caused by electrosomg remains)	Adequate effect	Often inadequate effect	Adequate effect only in protective structure below XEPS plate	Adequate effect only in protective structure below cellular glass plate	Adequate effect only in the protective structure beneath the cork plate
Reduction of Per-Sha 51 and Per-Sha 61 (above fault zones)	Adequate effect	Adequate effect when placed in side wall of appropriate cube system, otherwise often inadequate	Often inadequate effect	Often inadequate effect	Adequate effect
Reduction of Per-Sha through satellite dishes	Adequate effect	Adequate effect when placed in side wall of appropriate cube system, otherwise often inadequate	Inadequate effect	Inadequate effect	Inadequate effect

The Effect of the Feng Shui Power Disc 99 on Other Feng Shui Problems in the House

The Form School of feng shui is not only concerned with landscape forms or the forms of nature, but also with the effect of forms within the house. An entire series of Form School problems in the house require the space of the 0.67-Centimeter System or both of the 0.95 Centimeter Diagonal Systems A and B to have an impact. Other problems result from weakening of the aura of the house. Among other things, the Feng Shui Power Disc 99 causes an inactivation of the 0.67-Centimeter System or the two 0.95-Centimeter Diagonal Systems, as well as a strengthening of the house aura. As a result, this clears away a large number of the problems in the house. Please be aware that neither the described arrangement of the silica discs nor the XEPS plates, cellular glass plates, or cork tiles are capable of doing this. In the following section, we briefly describe inauspicious Form School situations for which the Feng Shui Power Disc 99 provides a good remedy or improvement. Within this context, we also provide some advice regarding the observed problems in these inauspicious feng shui situations.

Inauspicious Feng Shui Situations in the Bedroom

- **A door points to the bed**: This can result in the inexplicable weakening of the healthy constitution
- **A bed between two bedroom doors**: In addition to the situation described above, opposing doors can also have an irritating effect on the mental aspects of a human being.
- The **edges and corners of furniture** that point to the bed also have an unfavorable effect
- **Ceiling beams above the bed**: If there is a lengthwise beam above the middle of the marriage bed, this can cause or intensify problems related to separation. When the **lengthwise beam** is directly above one of the sleeping people, health problems may develop for this person because of an impairment of the aura function, similar to that described for the door that points to the bed. **Crosswise beams** above the sleeping person could cause health problems, particularly in the area of the body that has the crosswise beam above it.
- **Triangular windows** bring a great amount of unrest into the bedroom, for example. People who sleep in such a room report an increase in nightmares and other sleep disorders.

A Woman Repeatedly Asked for Advice from Her Feng Shui Consultant

A woman did not feel well in her spacious attic apartment. She slept poorly, couldn't concentrate when she did the housework, and felt considerably better when she was outside her apartment. She hoped a feng shui consultation would bring an improvement. All of the windows in the attic apartment were triangular. The feng shui consultant advised here to undertake a series of feng shui remedies. Cost reasons prevented her from having the windows altered. One after the other, she gradually put the rest of the recommended remedies into effect. However, the woman's complaints did not improve substantially. She contacted the consultant a number of times to discuss further feng shui remedies. Even then, there was not adequate improvement. So the feng shui consultant recommended the use of a Feng Shui Power Disc. After one week, there was a considerable improvement. After two more weeks, the woman felt well in her apartment for the first time.

Inauspicious Feng Shui Situations Outside of the House

- **Straight paths that lead to the house** can cause nervousness and sleep disorders in the house occupants. People who are generally so inclined will get silly ideas and tend to make more poor decisions. Curved paths to the house door are more auspicious.
- **Houses at T-crossings** display the same phenomenon.
- **Water that flows toward or away from the house** has an effect similar to that of straight paths that lead to the house.
- **Roof ridges from a neighboring house** that point to the entrance or a window can trigger feelings of fear in the occupants or even lead to a certain coldness. In addition, they reduce the protective function of the human aura.
- **Wind-tunnel effect:** A small gap between two houses that points at the house door creates the so-called wind-tunnel effect. The effect is similar to that of the roof ridges, but it may be even more intense.
- **Secret arrows (*An Jian*):** The Chinese give the name of secret arrows (*An Jian* in Chinese) to influences that emanate from building corners, roof ridges, or other sharp parts of a building with a straight direction of effect. These arrows are called "secret" because their course between the starting point, such as a building corner, and its arrival at the other building are invisible, even to people who are clairvoyant. The secret arrow generally opens the house up to inauspicious influences. Mirror facades can also trigger secret arrows to the neighboring buildings.

Inauspicious Feng Shui Situations for the Entrance Area of the House

- **A branchless tree or post in front of the entrance door** diminishes the flow of favorable energies into the house and opens the house up for inauspicious influences.
- **Lengthwise beams behind the front door** can trigger nervousness, poor decisions, and "silly thoughts" in the house occupants.
- **Crosswise beams behind the front door** can trigger feelings of fear or a certain coldness in house occupants in some cases.
- **A mirror directly opposite the front door** can open the house to inauspicious influences from the outside, depending on its dimensions and certain directional influences.
- **The corner of a wall directly opposite the front door** can have an inauspicious influence similar to that of a mirror.

Inauspicious Feng Shui Situations in the House

- **Long passageways in the house** can lead to nervousness and sleep disorders in the house occupants. People who are so inclined will have "silly thoughts" and tend to make poor decisions. This may also lead to feelings of fear and a certain coldness.
- **L-shaped rooms:** The best form for a room is a square. With a few exceptions, L-shaped and other non-rectangular rooms are inauspicious. We find increased inauspicious energies in an L-shaped room. For a bedroom, this means that a person may not feel like he or she has had enough sleep in the morning. For a living room, this may mean that a peaceful feeling does not arise there very easily. In a study, it may be more difficult to concentrate.
- **When the corners of a room are not at a right angle** but have an angle of less than 90 degrees, this is inauspicious. Spending time in such corners will increase the tendency toward concentration problems and making errors. Disinclination toward work may arise.
- **Staggered levels in a house** have a disruptive effect on the distribution of auspicious energies in the house.
- **Rooms with different ceiling heights** have more inauspicious energies, as already described for L-shaped rooms.
- **Toilets and drain pipes in the house** can lead to disruptions in the communication of the house occupants with each other. This may result in the people in the house talking less with each other and having less desire for contacts outside the house. The disinclination toward certain activities may increase, such as using leisure

time for hobbies. People feel more easily offended. Fits of crying also occur more frequently in children.

It is particularly **inauspicious** to have the toilet:

Above, below, or next to (especially to the right of) the front door

Above, below, or behind the bed

Above, below, or behind the kitchen stove

Above the dining room or study.

The inauspicious effect is usually the strongest when the toilet is above one of the rooms listed here. The effect is somewhat less when the toilet is beneath one of these rooms. If the toilet is next to one of these rooms, the effect is not particularly auspicious, but it is the most tolerable of these possibilities.

- **Chimney and fireplace:** In Europe, the chimney has traditionally been the focus of attention as an entrance possibility for undesirable influences. The undesirable influences can reach the lower floors in particular through the open fireplaces. This may lead to the occupants having difficulty in thinking straight. Furthermore, this may even lead to psychological disorders.
- **Air-conditioning systems and vent pipes:** Similar to chimneys and fireplaces, air-conditioning systems and vent pipes can lead to a distribution of undesired influences in the house.
- **Slanted roofs:** In rooms with a slanted roof exceeding about 22 degrees (to the horizontal plane), we find inauspicious influences similar to those described under chimney and fireplace. The effect is also intensified when the slant of the roof is more than 30 degrees and the top story has not been completed as living space.
- **Satellite dishes on the roof and the house wall:** In rooms beneath or next to satellite dishes, Per-Sha is not the only negative energy created. There will also be an increase in restlessness, and occupants have reported a sense of unwellness.
- **Fountains on the property or in the house:** Problems occur when the fountains when an inner diameter of about 1 1/2 feet (50 cm). There may be an increase in the dysregulation of the body, as well as accidents.
- **Ghost paths:** The Chinese give the name of ghost paths to the subtle and non-material paths that lead through a piece of property and bring inauspicious influences for its residents. Such paths are described as connecting two cemeteries, for example.

Chapter 6

Negative Impact of Electrosmog and Chemicals

Feng Shui and Electrosmog

No Previous Reliable Data on Threshold Value

The triumphant advance of electrotechnology in the private, business, and public sectors began at the end of the 19th century. This has brought us a great number of conveniences, yet only now have possible problems for our health increasingly come to the limelight. Construction biologists and biological electrotechnicians are attempting on the basis of physically measured data to work out threshold values meant to guarantee a tolerance level for human beings. In the process, an entire series of data is being gathered, such as the strengths of the electrical and magnetic fields, etc. It is difficult, particularly because of the complex influences, to comprehend the effects on human beings. Reliable data about threshold values that would guarantee safety has not been adequately presented.

Influence on Subtle Energies

It should be taken into consideration that both the electrical installations within the home, as well as the technical equipment of the power-supply companies such as long-distance transmission lines and transformer stations, the overhead wires of the railways, and the broadcasting and radar stations can influence the subtle energies that we examine in feng shui. Our fundamental opinion is that whatever can be measured in the physical sense should be. However, it is additionally necessary to determine the subtle influences with the tensor.

Complaints and Health Disorders Because of Electrosmog

A series of complaints and health disorders have been observed when people suffer negative effects because of electrosmog. Among these are:
• Headaches
• Decrease in physical and mental powers
• Fatigue
• Spells of dizziness

- Falling asleep only when extremely tired
- Light, superficial sleep
- General weakness
- States of exhaustion
- Functional disorders of the central nervous system
- Lack of concentration
- Tendency to sweat
- Cardiovascular disorders

EEG changes and changes in the blood picture have also been described.

Many Things Are Quite Obvious

During the feng shui inspections, many of the above-mentioned electrotechnical installations such as high-tension power lines, transformer stations, overhead wires of the railway, etc., immediately catch the eye; other problems are electricity meters and fuse-boxes next to the bedroom in the home, electrical cabling (particularly at the head of the bed), and electrical devices like television sets in the bedroom. In the following section, we will combines this negative impact under the term of electrosmog. As already described under Geo-Sha and Trans-Sha, the negative effects during sleep create the greatest problems in terms of electrosmog as well.

Orientation Measurements for Negative Impacts of Electrical Installations

If you are uncertain in dealing with electricity, then get the help of an electrician. When examining the sleeping area, it has proved effective to evaluate the negative impact of electrical installations in the household, at least for orientation purposes. The line voltage in the home is about 110 volts. For the purposes of orientation, it is possible to measure how much alternating voltage there is on the body in the sleeping area. This process is also called **capacitive coupling**. We would like to briefly introduce this procedure:

The orientating measurement of the negative impact of the electrical installations in the sleeping area is done with a so-called multimeter. A multimeter is an economical and popular electrotechnical measuring device with which alternating and direct-current voltage, alternating currents, etc., can be measured.

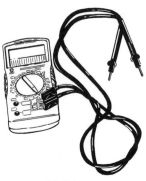

Multimeter

However, in this case only the function of measuring the alternating current voltage is used. At the same time, a measurement in the millivolt range must also be possible in order to receive an adequately precise measurement result. The following description is only intended for people who have enough experience in dealing with electrical installations in the household. Others should by all means leave the measuring procedure described here to an expert. Here is the technical procedure:

1) Find a ground connection. It is usually possible to use the ground of the wall socket (the lowest of the three openings in the wall socket). Then use the multimeter to check whether the wall socket is grounded. First use the two cables of the multimeter to determine whether there is alternating current voltage on the wall socket (generally 110 volts in the USA). Then measure the current-carrying socket of the wall socket against the grounding of the wall socket. If the wall socket is grounded correctly, the multimeter will also show an alternating current of about 110 volts.

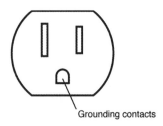

Grounding contacts

2) Now turn down the measuring range and measure it between the test person, who is lying on the sleeping area, and the grounding

of the wall socket. Turn the measuring range down one step at a time until you find an adequate sensitivity. If necessary, the contact between the test person and the multimeter can be improved by having the person touch a hand electrode or just a copper plate from which the alternating current is being measured.

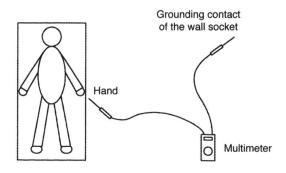

Measuring the alternating-current voltage on the body.

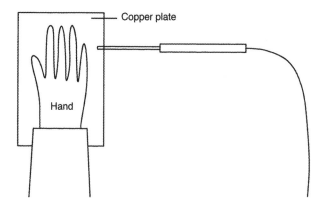

Measuring the alternating-current voltage on the body
(hand on the copper plate).

Values beneath 100 mV of alternating-current voltage are best. When the values are higher (for example, several thousand millivolts), you can turn off one or more electrical circuits at the fuse-box to determine whether a **demand switch** would bring sufficient improvement and which electrical circuits should be included with it. In the process, proceed in such a way that the fuse or circuit-breaker of the electrical circuit that supplies the bedroom is turned off first. If an adequate lowering of the measuring value does not occur, turn off further fuses (for example, in the adjoining bathroom) until you have determined which fuses need to be switched off in order to create an adequate lowering of the measuring value. These fuses can then be adjusted by an electrician using a demand switch. A demand switch only permits 3 to 4 volts of current on the lines of the respective electrical circuit, as long as no power-consuming devices are switched on. If a power-consuming device is turned on (for example, the ceiling lights, the nightstand lamp, etc.), the demand switch once again permits the usual current of 110 volts in the supply mains. There is also a demand switch with an adjustable threshold value, above which the 110 volts of alternating current once again enter the supply mains. This can prevent power-consuming devices that are connected so they initially only use very little electricity when they are switched on (such as vacuum cleaners) from activating the demand switch, thereby permitting the full current in the mains. In this simple way, you can make sure that there is only a minor strain on the sleeping person during the night.

The demand switch only functions (with "function" meaning that it switches the current in the electrical circuits behind it to somewhere between 3 and 4 volts) when no **"secret power-consumers"** are switched on. For example, secret power-consumers are cassette recorders, radios and other devices that have a transformer on the inside or even at the beginning of the cable (which you can recognize by the cube-shaped plug that often just has a thin cable leading to the device itself). The transformer consumes minor amounts of energy, even when the accompanying device is not operating. You can frequently recognize this because the transformer always feels a bit warm. If the transformer consumes electricity, this naturally means that there is a 110 volt alternating current on the electrical circuit. In this case, the demand switch would not create any protection for the sleeping person.

35,000 Millivolts in a Child's Sleeping Area
A 7-year-old girl, who had been prematurely born, suffered from a whole series of health complaints. These included asthma and a susceptibility to infections. During the feng shui examination, it became obvious that

the girl's sleeping area was subject to 35,000 millivolts (=35 volts) of alternating current. The parents were advised to have the electrical installation of the house checked by an electrician. This resulted in the discovery that a technical error had been causing this high level of negative impact. The error was eliminated so that the girl could once again sleep without disturbances.

Here are some further examples of the technical procedure in practice:

You Already Achieve the Threshold Value with a Demand Switch for the Bedroom

You find a strain of 2,500 millivolts on the test person in the sleeping area. After switching off the fuse for the bedroom, this value sinks to 95 millivolts. We can assume that the negative impact in the sleeping area will be distinctly reduced when the electrical circuit that supplies the bedroom is provided with a demand switch. This switch can be installed by an electrician.

What Do You Do If You Do Not Reach the Desired Threshold Value?

The negative impact on the sleeping area is 3,500 millivolts. Turning off the fuse for the bedroom only brings this down to 800 millivolts. Additionally turning off the fuse for the adjoining bathroom reduces the value to 200 millivolts. A further reduction cannot be achieved by switching off any other electrical circuits in the house. A negative electromagnetic impact is sometimes also created by neighbors who live next to, as well as below or above the examined residence. Since it usually is not easy to include the neighbors' electrical installations in a demand switch and there is also no way of checking whether or not the neighbor has a "secret power-consumer" attached even after a demand switch has been installed, the **individual threshold value** of the capacitive coupling can initially be determined by using a tensor or pendulum. You should ask: "**Is the individual threshold value of ... (name of person) above 100 millivolts?**"

If you get a YES, then continue to ask: "... **above 200 millivolts?**," "... **above 300 millivolts?**," etc., until you receive a NO. If, for example, you receive a YES for "... **above 300 millivolts?**" and a NO **for** "... **above 400 millivolts?**," the individual threshold value lies between 300 and 400 millivolts. A strain of 200 millivolts, as given in the example, would therefore be tolerable and you would not have to take any further measures. In this example, a device to automatically regulate the power level for the bedroom and bathroom would be installed by an electrician.

When the Wall Socket Is Not Grounded

If you discover that the wall socket is not grounded because you do not measure the expected 110 volts between the current-carrying wall socket and the grounding of the wall socket with the multimeter, you can then attempt, for example, to use the central heating as the ground. The multimeter will confirm an adequate ground for this purpose if about 110 volts of alternating current are shown between the current-carrying wall socket and the central heating. Now measure the capacitive coupling between the test person and the central heating as a ground. As an alternative to this, you can also attempt to find a ground to measure with through an extension cable from another room. If you do not have adequate grounding, the multimeter will not give you the data you need for this purpose in order to compare with the desired values of 100 millivolts, for example.

Measuring the Capacitive Coupling Is Only Suitable for Assessing the Negative Impact of Electrical Installations in the Household

We want to expressly emphasize that the method described here of measuring the capacitive coupling is only an orientational measurement of the negative impact of electrical installations in the household. This method is completely unsuitable for evaluating the negative effects because of directional radio antennas, high-tension power lines, transformer stations, or overhead wires of a railway in the vicinity of the house. If there is a reasonable suspicion that these installations lead to a negative impact, a specialist (such as a biological electrotechnician) should be consulted for evaluating the negative impact with his or her measuring methods. In addition to this, you may possibly have to determine the influence on the subtle energies, particularly on the Vital-Qi (which we will soon discuss here) by using the tensor.

It is better not to have television sets and computers located in the bedroom. There are also other effects that cannot be assessed by measuring the capacitive coupling. In this context, there is a definite problem in bedrooms that have one corner set up as a private office with a computer (along with an Internet connection, for example).

Be Careful of Technical Shielding Measures Using Metal

In case the biological electrotechnician recommends shielding measures such as Mumetal (metal foil that cannot be magnetized and therefore lets no magnetic fields pass through it), be sure that the metal brings no additional Trans-Sha into the bedroom. In addition, check to see whether there is an influence on the subtle energies that has evaded the technical measurement. It is possible that, despite adequate shielding of a technical sort, the influence on the subtle energies is still so strong that the sleeping area must be moved somewhere else.

Some Comments About Electrical Lighting

It is good to have rooms adequately illuminated. We advise against the use of halogen lamps if they are, as usual, operated with alternating current. Like fluorescent tubes, they produce a flickering that is invisible to the eye yet still very irritating to it. This flickering goes on and off 60 times a second. In addition, the common transformer-operated halogen lamps create a strong electromagnetic field. Normal filament bulbs do not flicker, even when operated with alternating current, since the filament is too inert.

Negative Chemical Effects

It is even more difficult to discuss this topic than that of electrosmog within the scope of this book. On the one hand, there is an enormous number of chemical compounds that can create a negative impact in the home; on the other hand, the spectrum of chemical compounds that create a negative impact is constantly changing. Some compounds are prohibited, and others that are initially considered safe take their place. After several years, it then turns out that the new compounds also cause health problems, possibly of a different type require and other ways of finding evidence of them.

If You Suspect a Negative Chemical Effect, Get the Advice of a Specialist

If you suspect that there is a negative chemical effect in your home, then get the advice of a specialist. In addition to taking samples or measurements on site is the experience that professionals have gathered during their long years of work. For example, just naming the construction date of a certain prefabricated house is often enough to get on the track of a specific wood preservative. In addition, especially since a part of the analysis, as well as the renovation measures in particular, are very expensive in this area, professional competence and adequate experience are necessary.

The Threshold Values Alone Are Not Sufficient for People Who Have Suffered Strain for Years

One problem is that people who were exposed to a certain negative impact for years react with a sensitization so that, even when the negative impact in the house has fallen below the customary threshold value, the affected person still distinctly reacts to certain negative chemical effects. This can even lead to a general oversensitivity to chemicals. Furthermore, it has been observed that in negatively affected houses, the people who show the most symptoms are the ones who are exposed to the strain the longest during the day. So the adult who stays primarily in the home during the day is most frequently affected the most, followed by small children who spend a great deal of time in the house, but the person who is employed displays less symptoms if he or she spends the greater part of the day outside the home.

Solvents

One of the substance groups that create problems is that of solvents. For example, solvents are found in chipboard (and therefore also in furniture) in the form of formaldehyde, but they are also used in gluing carpets. The existence of formaldehyde and other solvents in the room air can be proved. Before having a sample taken, be sure that the room has not been aired beforehand for the defined amount of time since just a relatively minor amount of solvent can be proved in the room air shortly after it has been thoroughly aired.

Wood Preservatives

The health problems related to the use of wood preservatives inside the home have now become more obvious to the general public. Many people had suffered from intense health disorders as a result of wood preservative that had been initially declared safe for use inside the home. Many of the wood preservatives used in earlier times, like pentachlorphenol (PCP) are now prohibited. In the meantime, the so-called pyrethroids that can be found in almost all wool rugs and wool carpets are quite widespread. Even if you do not have small children who play on the floor, you should still consider doing without these products. In terms of the negative effects caused by chemical substances, synthetic carpets may be safer than wool carpets with a high pyrethroid content. The negative impact because of wood preservatives can be estimated on the basis of the concentration of these substances in wood samples. The concentration of the pyrethroids is determined in the household dust.

Heavy Metals

The problem with heavy metals has clearly declined since lead pipes are no longer used as water pipes. Lead pipes in old houses are usually coated with lime on the inside so that hardly any lead is released. There are occasionally problems with copper because of copper pipes.

Chapter 7

The "Five Elements" and the Aura of the House

Wu Xing: The Five Laws of Change

When the Europeans began to more intensively examine Chinese culture at the end of the 19th Century, they attempted to compare or link Chinese ideas with those of the West. The four elements of air, fire, water, and earth were familiar in the West. When taking a superficial look at these ideas, some Western researchers thought there was a connection or correlation of these four elements with the Chinese Five Laws of Change. Wu Xing was therefore often translated as the "Five Elements" in the West. Although we now know that the four elements of Greek philosophy cannot be directly compared with the Wu Xing, the translation of the "Five Elements" (or also the "Five Qualities") has continued up to this day. However, in the following we want to stay with the Chinese term of Wu Xing or the English translation of the "Five Laws of Change" in order to prevent misunderstandings.

The Five Laws of Change, Wu Xing, are five related mechanisms from the 5th dimension that have an effect on various energies, carriers, and structures of the 3rd dimension. In a certain sense, these are the natural laws* of the 5th dimension. The individual Laws of Change have a very specific interaction with each other. They influence our health, our mental functions, our moods, and astrological circumstances.

The Chinese have given the Five Laws of Change the names of materials that activate each respective Law of Change (transformational mechanisms).

In Chinese, these materials are called:
- **Mu** (Wood)
- **Huo** (Fire)
- **Tu** (Earth)
- **Jin** (Metal, actually Gold)
- **Shui** (Water)

---

* The Five Laws of Change have an effect on our 3rd dimension that is just as real as the laws of nature known from physics, such as gravity and electromagnetism.

The Meaning of the Five Laws
of Change for Our Health

In its diagnostics and therapy, as well as in the interplay of yin and yang, Traditional Chinese Medicine is also based on the Five Laws of Change. Through the Five Laws of Change, there is the possibility of exerting influence on all physical and mental functions. In addition to balanced nutrition and the corresponding physical-mental activities, the qualities of energies in the room are very significant.

Materials Activate the Five Laws of Change

Feng shui analyzes the qualities of the various energies in the room with relation to the Five Laws of Change and shows a series of possibilities for influencing these energy qualities. Among other things, this is possible through certain **materials.** The proper use of these materials brings our bodily functions back into equilibrium. Our mental functions are also influenced and supported in a positive manner as a result.

The energies in the room are normally present in all five Wu Xing qualities. However, the individual qualities may exist to greatly varying degrees at the same time. But individual people and certain activities frequently require a different proportion of Wu Xing qualities. We can influence this: When a certain energy quality needs to be strengthened in a room, we can bring the material suited for this purpose into the room. We would first like to give you an overview of the suitable materials and their types of effects.

How the Material Wood Activates the Wood Law of Change

When we additionally bring an object of wood into a room, the **Wood Law of Change** starts becoming active. The **wood energy quality** is strengthened. Clairvoyant people notice a green fog around the added object. The Chinese therefore classify the **color green** with the energy quality of wood.

How Fire Activates the Fire Law of Change

When we light a fire in a room (for example, as the flame of a candle or a fireplace), the **Fire Law of Change** starts becoming active. In this case, the **energy quality of fire** is intensified. Clairvoyant people see this energy quality in the red color. Logically enough, the Chinese have also classified the **color red** with the energy quality of fire.

How the Material Earth Activates the Earth Law of Change

When we additionally bring earth into a room, the **Earth Law of Change** starts becoming active. The **earth energy quality** is strengthened. Clairvoyant people see this energy quality in a yellowish to light-brown color. The Chinese therefore classify the **color yellow** with the energy quality of earth.

How the Material Metal Activates the Metal Law of Change

When we additionally bring an object of metal into a room, the **Metal Law of Change** starts becoming active. In this case, the **metal energy quality** has been increased. Clairvoyant people see this energy quality in a whitish color. The Chinese therefore classify the **color white** with the energy quality of metal.

How Water Activates the Water Law of Change

If water is additionally brought into a room, the **Water Law of Change** starts becoming active. The **water energy quality** is now strengthened. Clairvoyant people see this energy quality in a blue color. The Chinese therefore classify the **color blue** with the energy quality of water.

Other Materials Also Activate the Laws of Change

In the following section, we want to go into more detail about the materials that have given the respective Laws of Change their names. In addition to these, there are further materials that also activate the Laws of Change. As of now, we want to give the name of transformational materials to both types of materials. **Transformational materials** can be specifically used when building a house to more intensely emphasize certain qualities. In the finished house, interior-decoration objects or even ornaments can be consciously placed and thereby also adjusted to the current conditions at any time. When using the transformational materials, it is important to know that almost all transformational materials made or processed by human beings have a limited "life span." This means that they can only activate the respective Law of Change for a limited time.

Wood as a Transformational Material

Particularly in earlier times, a great deal of wood was used in the construction of a house. Even today, there are frequently window frames, door frames, floors, ceiling and wall linings, as well as roof frameworks, made of solid wood. Interior furnishings like chairs, tables, and shelves are either completely or partially made of wood. Furthermore, things like statues, other types of wood carvings, bowls, little boxes, and even wicker baskets are made of wood. Cork also activates the Wood Law of Change. Chipboard is at least partially made of wood.

Living plants, drapes or floor covering made of cotton or other plant fibers also activate the Wood Law of Change. Dried plants and ornamental gourds, books and magazines, fruit, or baked goods can activate the Wood Law of Change, at least for a time.

Life Span of Wood Transformational Materials
- Wood: 40 years
- Wood parquet: 40 years
- Cork parquet: 40 years
- Wicker baskets: 5 to 7 years
- Drapes or floor coverings of cotton or other plant fibers: approx. 2 years
- Chipboard: approx. 2 years
- Dried plants and ornamental gourds: approx. 1 year
- Books and magazines: 1 year (a place for current magazines that are replaced on a regular basis would basically be suited for a longer period of time since the limitations of time would be neutralized in this case)

Fire as a Transformational Material
Today, we rarely find open fire in interior rooms.

However, the Fire Law of Change is also activated by sheet glass (not blown glass). For example, sheet glass is used in panes of windows, doors, closets, and glass-covered pictures. Sheet glass is also used for shelves, tabletops, and as a covering for tables and cupboards.

Sheet glass in mirrors is combined with metal and, when evaluating its effect, always take the additional metal into consideration. In addition, the mirror dimensions, as well as possible problems created by Trans-Sha because of the metal portions, should be considered. The same dimensions as for front doors (see the section on *Perm-Qi* on page 111) apply to mirror dimensions. You can find further details under the keyword of *Mirror* in the glossary of the appendix on page 221.

Life Span of Fire Transformational Materials
- Pebbles: practically unlimited
- Sheet glass: 20 to 45 years
- Sheet glass: approx. 20 years in mirrors
- Candle flames and fireplaces: as long as they burn

Earth as a Transformational Material

Included under the transformational materials of earth is potting soil, although plant remnants may additionally represent the transformational materials of wood.

Other materials that activate the Earth Law of Change are natural stone, bricks, and concrete. However, please pay attention to the metal portion of reinforced concrete with rebar. Crystals (gemstones), porcelain, ceramics, wool, leather and/or furs, and synthetics belong in this category.

Synthetics are used in many ways in modern interior decoration. Also pay attention to things like the plastic coating of furniture.

Life Span of Earth Transformational Materials
- Crystals (gemstones): unlimited
- Natural stones: practically unlimited
- Porcelain: 80 to 110 years
- Bricks: 80 years
- Leather and furs: 50 to 60 years
- Ceramics: 50 years
- Reinforced concrete with rebar: 30 years
- Wool rugs and other wool textiles: 30 years
- Synthetics: 20 to 25 years*
- Natural silk: 10 to 20 years
- Stearin candles: 2 years
- Beeswax: 1 year

Metal as a Transformational Material

Metals of all types belong among the transformational materials of metal. Gold has the strongest effect. In addition to "metal," the Chinese term *Jin* can also be translated as "gold." A great deal of

---

* Synthetically coated furniture made on a base of chipboard is solely a ground transformational material after an age of about 2 years.

metal has been used in both house construction and interior decoration for a number of decades now.

Please be extremely careful with the placement of metals, particularly in the sleeping area, since serious health disorders frequently occur because of Trans-Sha. This also applies to the placement of mirrors, which represent the transformational material of metal and fire (because of the sheet glass). We generally advise against hanging mirrors in the sleeping area.

Life Span of Metal Transformational Materials
- Gold bars: approx. 120 years
- Gold rings: approx. 80 to 90 years
- Steel: 25 to 50 years
- Iron: 40 years
- Brass: 35 years
- Lead: 25 years
- Aluminum: 14 years
- Mercury (for example, in thermometers): 12 years
- Copper: 11 years
- Bronze: 10 years
- Mirror coating: approx. 9 years
- Silver: 6 to 10 years

Water as a Transformational Material

The ideal transformational material of water is water itself, especially in its swirling form (as a fountain, for example). Water that does not move can also activate the Water Law of Change, at best when it is not covered.

Furthermore, the Water Law of Change is activated through blown glass (drinking glasses, glass bowls, glass vases, glass figurines, and the like).

Life Span of Water Transformational Materials
- Blown glass: approx. 20 years

The Aura of the House and Its Structures

The Outer Aura Structures

Like the human being, the house also has an aura: this is divided into two outer hulls. The hulls have a protective function for the house and the occupants. The complete development of the house's aura only takes place starting at a certain house size. The minimum volume of the house for this purpose must be at least 180 cubic meters (about 235 cubic yards), with a minimum height and minimum width of approx. 14 feet (4 m).

The thickness of these hulls and their distance from the house is independent of the floor space and height of the house, which means that the following dimensions remain constant. We find (seen from within) the first hull at a distance of about 4 feet (130 cm) to about 5 1/2 feet (170 cm) from the house, giving it a thickness of about 1 1/2 feet (40 cm). We find the second hull at 10 feet (310 cm) to 15 feet (440 cm), which means that it is approx. 4 feet (130 cm) thick. In concrete houses, the hulls may be shifted between 12 and 16 inches (30 and 40 cm) with respect to the outside.

These hulls are not only found around the side walls of the house, but also beneath the house and including the cellar, if there is one. The downward distance from the floor of the cellar for the first hull is then also about 4 feet (130 cm) to about 5 1/2 feet (170 cm) and 10 feet (310 cm) to 15 feet (440 cm) for the second hull, taking into consideration the special characteristics of concrete as described above.

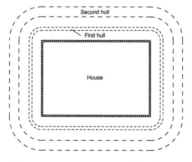

Outer aura structures of the house.

Inner Aura Structures

Within its interior, the aura of the house possesses certain structures that are important for both the distribution as well as the absorbability of energies and information. The aura of the human being is connected with this inner aura structure. The **mental portion** of the human being not only moves within the aura of the person, but also within the structures of the house's inner aura.

Among other things, we find a **sector-shaped structure**, the sectors of which extend outward to the first hull of the aura.

Sector-Shaped Aura Structure

A spatial, star-shaped structure with 48 sectors (somewhat like the pieces of a cake) are formed in the interior of the house. Each of them possesses the same angle size. These sectors extend from the center in the shape of a star to the inner hull of the house. The area within which the mind aspect of the human being moves includes the house's entire sector-shaped inner aura structure.

The sectors are important for the distribution and absorbability of the energies and information in the house. In the process, several neighboring sectors are used in the same way according to various criteria. The type of distribution and the absorbability of the energies and information has an influence upon our health, our family life, as well as our economic success and spiritual growth. In this book, we want to deal with the sectors that are important for our health. Further aspects of the house's aura structure will be discussed in subsequent volumes.

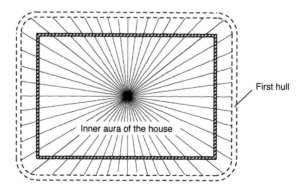

The sector-shaped aura structure consists of 48 sectors.

The Projection of the Sectors onto the Floor Plan of the House

When the floor plan of the house is not a square, it is adjusted to form an imaginary square. From the center of this square, the sectors are projected onto the floor plan of the house.

If we look at a house in spatial terms, we must alter the shape of houses that are not a right parallelepiped, so that the form of the house is that of an imaginary parallelepiped so that all the parts of the house can be found within the parallelepiped.

The central point from which the sectors project onto the floor plan of the individual stories then lies in the center of the right parallelepiped in which the entire house is found.

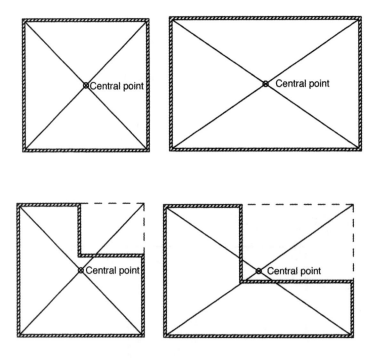

The central point within the sector-shaped aura structure in the house is the central point of the square or rectangular floor plan. In the case of left-out spaces, the floor plan is extended to create a square or rectangle.

Chapter 8

The Eight Trigram Sectors

The Eight Trigrams and Their Sectors

The **eight trigram sectors** are particularly important for a human being's health. Six sectors each of the house's inner aura structure are combined here as a unit. The eight trigram sectors each cover an angle of 45 degrees. Their center is oriented toward approx. 2.6 degrees west of the main and intermediate geographic directions. This means that the center of the trigram section Kan is oriented toward the feng shui direction of north. The geographic direction of north is generally found on site maps, city maps, and other maps. Each trigram is assigned to a trigram sector.

The eight trigrams are derived from the principle of **yin** and **yang**. The Chinese traditionally use horizontal lines to illustrate yin and yang. A solid horizontal line symbolizes yang, and an interrupted line symbolizes yin. (We have given a brief description of the qualities of yin and yang at the beginning of Chapter 4, on page 105.) The eight trigrams are made of a combination of three horizontal lines respectively. The distribution of the eight trigrams into the above-mentioned sectors of the inner aura structure of the house is also called **Bagua**.

The Eight Trigrams and Their Sectors (Overview)

Trigrams	Sector* in the House	Direction
Kan	334.9–19.9 degrees	North
Gen	19.9–64.5 degrees	Northeast
Zhen	64.9–109.9 degrees	East
Sun	109.9–154.9 degrees	Southeast
Li	154.9–199.9 degrees	South
Kun	199.9–244.9 degrees	Southwest
Dui	244.9–289.9 degrees	West
Qian	289.9–334.9 degrees	Northwest

---

* The stated degree figure refers the geographic direction of north.

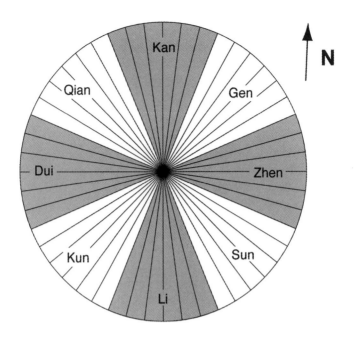

The eight trigrams and their sectors (chart to copy in appendix on page 241).

In addition to the classification of the directions or sectors with the eight trigrams, each trigram is also associated with one of the Five Laws of Change (Wu Xing). Furthermore, the Traditional Chinese Medicine recognizes the relationships between acupuncture meridians, Wu Xing, and the eight trigrams. On the basis of these relationships, a tendency toward a certain health disorder can result in one trigram sector for a certain group of people. It should also be mentioned at this point that the Feng Shui Power Disc 99 reduces the absorption of harmful energies by the human aura in the individual trigram sectors below a critical threshold.

The Eight Trigrams and Their Relationship to the Directions and Wu Xing

Kan

The trigram Kan consists of (always seen from above to below) an interrupted line, a solid line, and an interrupted line.

Wu Xing: Water
Meridian: Kidneys, Bladder

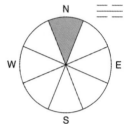

Sector of the house: North

Gen

The trigram Gen consists of a solid line and two interrupted lines.

Wu Xing: Earth (soft)
Meridian: Stomach, spleen-pancreas

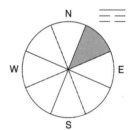

Sector of the house: Northeast

Zhen

The trigram Zhen consists of two interrupted lines and one solid line.

Wu Xing: Wood (hard)
Meridian: Circulation, triple warmer

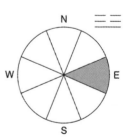

Sector of the house: East

Sun

The trigram Sun consists of two solid lines and one interrupted line.

Wu Xing: Wood (soft)
Meridian: Liver, gallbladder

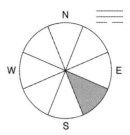

Sector of the house: Southeast

Li

The trigram Li consists of one solid line, one interrupted line, and one solid line.

Wu Xing: Fire
Meridian: Heart, small intestine

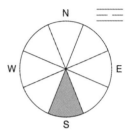

Sector of the house: South

Kun

The trigram Kun consists of three interrupted lines.

Wu Xing: Earth (hard)
Meridian: Governor and conception vessel

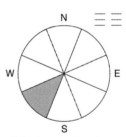

Sector of the house: Southwest

Dui

The trigram Dui consists of an interrupted line and two solid lines.

Wu Xing: Metal (soft)
Meridian: Large intestine, lungs

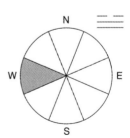

Sector of the house: West

Qian

The trigram Qian consists of three solid lines.

Wu Xing: Metal (hard)
Meridian: Governor and conception vessel

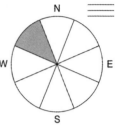

Sector of the house: northwest

Trigram Sectors Can Influence Your Health

In Western literature, much has been written about the psychological aspects of the Chinese animal signs. But here we are interested in the tangible health aspects that decide whether it is auspicious or inauspicious to sleep in a certain trigram sector.

The Chinese Animals Sign of the Year

Chinese astrology can help us determine which trigram sector may be problematic for our health. Special significance is placed upon the movement of the planet Jupiter in Chinese astrology. Jupiter moves once around the Sun in twelve years, which means it covers about one-twelfth of its path in one year. Each twelfth of its orbit around the Sun, and therefore each year, has an animal sign ascribed to it by the Chinese. These animal signs should not be confused with the Western signs of the Zodiac. The Chinese name the years according to the following animals:

- *Tiger*
- *Hare (or Rabbit)*
- *Dragon*
- *Snake*
- *Horse*
- *Ram (or Sheep)*

- *Monkey*
- *Cock*
- *Dog*
- *Wild Boar (or Pig)*
- *Rat*
- *Buffalo (or Ox)*

Chapter 9 page 207 ff *Discusses the animal signs of the year.*

The Chinese Animal Signs of the Month

The Chinese not only classify the same animal sign with years, but also with the months. They have two different methods of counting the months. The first is counting the twelve months (sections) within a solar year. The months are equally long here and always start with the same position of the Sun. For the other method, they also use the lunar calendar. This approach divides the year into twelve lunar months, whereby a "leap" month is added every two to three years according to a specific system. This is necessary since the length of time from one new moon to the next is only a little more than 29.5 days. The leap month is attributed to the same animal sign as the month before it.

How Do I Find My Chinese Animal Sign of the Month?

When you search for your Chinese animal sign of the lunar month, first look up your birth year in the tables of the appendix. Keep in mind that the Chinese lunar year does not start on January 1st like our Western year, but with the 2nd new moon after the Winter Solstice. This 2nd new moon after the Winter Solstice is also the beginning of the 1st Chinese lunar month of the year. The respective beginning dates for the lunar months of each respective year can also be found in the tables. So you can clearly assign a Chinese lunar month to your date of birth. If your date of birth is the first day of the Chinese lunar month, you should also consider your time of birth and compare to see the time at which the respective lunar month actually began.

Now you have used the lunar month of your birth to find your animal sign of the month. The next step is to correlate this animal sign with one of the eight trigrams. This is simple to do on the basis of the following table:

Chinese Animal Sign of the Lunar Month	Personal Trigram of the Lunar Month	Beginning of the Lunar Month in*
1st Tiger	Zhen	January or February
2nd Hare (or Rabbit)	Sun	February or March
3rd Dragon	Kun	March or April
4th Snake	Li	April or May

5th Horse	Li	May or June
6th Ram (or Sheep)	Women: Gen Men: Kun	June or July
7th Monkey	Qian	July or August
8th Cock	Dui	August or September
9th Dog	Kun	September or October
10th Wild Boar (or Pig)	Kan	October or November
11th Rat	Kan	November or December
12th Buffalo (or Ox)	Gen	December or January

If, for example, you were born in the month of the **Dragon**, your trigram is **Kun**. If you were born in the month of the Cock, your trigram is **Dui**. If you are female and born in the month of the **Ram**, your trigram is **Gen**; if you are male and born in the month of the **Ram**, your trigram is **Kun**.

You now have found your trigram using the animal sign of your birth month. You will certainly be interested in knowing how this trigram relates to the sleeping area that you have chosen.

Tendency Toward Certain Health Disorders

Approx. 12% of all people have, at least during certain age periods, a tendency to suffer from certain health disorders if they sleep in a trigram sector unfavorable for their health. This means that these people must be very careful about the sector of the house in which their bedroom is located. The unfavorable sectors can be determined on the basis of the personal trigram of the lunar month. Before we delve into which trigram sectors are inauspicious for a person with a certain personal trigram of the lunar month, we should first clarify whether or not the respective person is at all susceptible to illness (predispositioned) in such a trigram sector.

---

* The exact beginning and ending dates of the individual lunar months can be found in the table of the appendix on page 228 ff.

If you are confident in working with the tensor or pendulum, ask the concrete question: *"On the basis of my birth month, am I generally predispositioned to trigram-related health disorders if I sleep in one of the respective sectors?"*

If you receive a NO, you can also have your results checked by a second person, who should also be skilled and confident in working with the tensor or pendulum. The question would then be: *"Is ... (name) generally predispositioned to trigram-related health disorders if he/she sleeps in one of the respective sectors?"*

If this person also receives a NO, then you are not among the group of predispositioned people. According to this aspect, you can then have your bedroom in any of the trigram sectors. This means that you are among the 88% of the people who have no problems with this aspect of trigrams.

If you receive a YES, then continue with the next section.

Check to See Which Trigram Sector Is Unfavorable for You

You may take one or more sectors into consideration. The following list shows all the possible problematic sectors with the corresponding probability of illness for each personal trigram. In addition, each sector states whether women or men tend to be affected by it. The age group that is most likely to be affected by this respective illness is also included on the list. We will first explain the meaning of the individual categories:

Probability of illness: We have stated the probability of illness with the letters A to E. Using these letters, you can make the following estimations: Of the 100 people who become ill within this context:

50% become ill in the sector with the probability of A
20% become ill in the sector with the probability of B
13% become ill in the sector with the probability of C
10% become ill in the sector with the probability of D
7% become ill in the sector with the probability of E

Gender: Here you will find out whether women or men are more frequently affected. If it states women, this means that two-thirds of the affected are women and one-third are men. If it states men, this means the distribution is reversed, meaning two-thirds men and one-third women.

Age: Within this context, there is a differentiation between the various age groups:

    0) Unborn
    1) 0 to 16 years
    2) 16 to 32 years
    3) 32 to 48 years
    4) 48 to 65 years
    5) 65 and up

The statistics in a specific age group mean that of 100 persons who have become ill, 70% become ill in this age group, 20% in the section below, and 10% in the section above.

Health disorders: Since we cannot explain the basic principles of Traditional Chinese Medicine at this point, we have attempted to summarize the typical symptoms and feelings of ill-health. The individually occurring symptoms are frequently functional and do not always have a clinical picture that can be easily classified in the Western sense.

First look for your trigram in the following list. There you will find all the sectors listed that may possibly create problems. Ask about all of the sectors that could apply to you on the basis of your age. Be aware that in addition to the given age group, the age groups below and above could be affected as well.

The question is: *"Because of my birth month, am I predispositioned to sector-related illnesses if I sleep in the ... (trigram name) sector?"*

Ask about each individual sector and make note of the results.

Here as well, you can let the results be checked by another person who is skilled and confident at working with the tensor or pendulum. Then the question would be: *"Is ... (name) predispositioned to sector-related illnesses if he/she sleeps in the ... (trigram name) sector?"*

If you receive a YES for one or more sectors, you avoid this or these sectors in your house in terms of where you sleep if there you do not have a Feng Shui Power Disc 99 placed in your house.

If you are uncertain when asking these questions with the tensor or pendulum, to be on the safe side you can consider your trigram assignment when selecting your sleeping area as if you belong to the group of people who are predispositioned to it or use a Feng Shui Power Disc 99.

Depending upon the trigram that you have determined for your birth month, you can read the possible problem sectors on the following pages.

Trigram Kan (Birth Month Wild Boar or Rat)

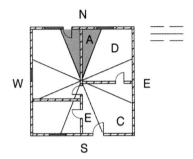

Sector Kan
Probability of illness: A
Gender: Male
Age: 16 to 32 years
Health Disorders: Pyelitis, nervous bladder, diseases of the external ear, ringing in the ears (not tinnitus), nail diseases

Sector Sun
Probability of illness: C
Gender: Male
Age: 32 to 48 years
Health Disorders: Intense trembling caused by cold, dryness in mouth, as well as general dryness of the mucous membranes and skin

Sector Gen
Probability of illness: D
Gender: Male
Age: 16 to 32 years
Health Disorders: Irritation of the periosteum

Sector Li
Probability of illness: E
Gender: Female
Age: 0 to 16 years
Health Disorders: Severe inflammation of middle ear with deafness

Trigram Gen (Birth Month Buffalo for Men and Women, as well as Ram for Women)

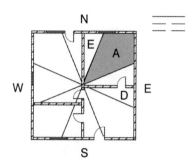

Sector Gen
Probability of illness: A
Gender: Male
Age: 0 to 16 years
Health Disorders: Stomach diseases (for example, weak stomach in infant)

Sector Zhen
Probability of illness: D
Gender: Male
Age: 0 to 16 years
Health Disorders: Diseases of the thymus gland, the male reproductive glands (for example, testicles drop too late into scrotum)

Sector Kan
Probability of illness: E
Gender: Female
Age: Related to unborn who would have had their time of birth in a Gen month
Health Disorders: Deformations of arms, legs, and muscles

Trigram Zhen (Birth Month Tiger)

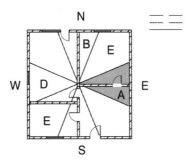

Sector Zhen
Probability of illness: A
Gender: Male
Age: 32 to 48 years
Health Disorders: Chronic irritation of neck lymph nodes

Sector Kan
Probability of illness: B
Gender: Male
Age: 32 to 48 years
Health Disorders: Diseases of bone marrow, nail diseases

Sector Dui
Probability of illness: D
Gender: Male
Age: 32 to 48 years
Health Disorders: Biliary tract diseases, intolerance of fat

Sector Kun
Probability of illness: E
Gender: Male
Age: 16 to 32 years
Health Disorders: Parodontosis, degenerative joint and tendon diseases (such as tendinitis), Shen disorders (including impaired memory)

Sector Gen
Probability of illness: E
Gender: Male
Age: 16 to 32 years

Health Disorders: Degenerative joint diseases, particularly of the hands (seen under the aspect of a Vata disorder in the Indian healing art of Ayurveda)

Trigram Sun (Birth Month Hare)

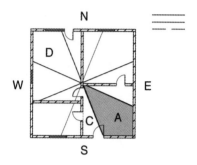

Sector Sun
Probability of illness: A
Gender: Female
Age: 32 to 48 years
Health Disorders: Liver diseases (tendency toward Hepatitis A, disorders of detoxification function, elevation of blood lipids cholesterol and triglyceride

Sector Li
Probability of illness: C
Gender: Female
Age: 48 to 65 years
Health Disorders: Impaired vision, retinopathy

Sector Qian
Probability of illness: D
Gender: Female
Age: 32 to 48 years
Health Disorders: Chronic ovaritis (inflammation of an ovary) and precursors

Trigram Li (Birth Month Snake or Horse)

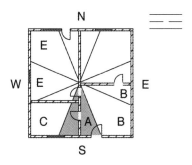

Sector Li
Probability of illness: Female
Gender: Female
Age: 16 to 32 years
Health Disorders: Cardiovascular disease (functional circulatory disorders like high and low blood pressure, as well as stroke), Shen disorders: speech disorders* (speaking too quickly or too slowly, frequent clearing of throat)

Sector Zhen
Probability of illness: B
Gender: Female
Age: 16 to 32 years
Health Disorders: Low blood pressure, Shen disorders (including poor orientation, problems in planning things, tendency toward muscle cramps)

Sector Sun
Probability of illness: B
Gender: Female
Age: 16 to 32 years
Health Disorders: Tendency toward flu diseases, vascular diseases (including thrombosis of the thighs)

Sector Kun
Probability of illness: C
Gender: Female
Age: 32 to 48 years

---

* In this case, speech disorders do not include stuttering.

Health Disorders: Increased menstruation, menstrual complaints at start of menopause, increased bleeding from the gums, disorders of Shen: including taste disorders, disorders of color perception and speech disorders* (for example, speaking too quickly or too slowly, frequent clearing of throat)

Sector Qian
Probability of illness: E
Gender: Male
Age: 0 to 16 years
Health Disorders: Fever (excessive fever reaction)

Sector Dui
Probability of illness: E
Gender: Female
Age: 0 to 16 years
Health Disorders: Irritation of the diaphragm (hiccups)

Trigram Kun (Birth Month Dragon or Dog for Men and Women, as well as Ram for Men)

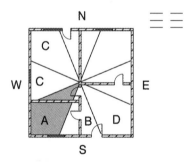

Sector Kun
Probability of illness: A
Gender: Female
Age: 48 to 65 years
Health Disorders: Gastrointestinal diseases, particularly: obstipation (constipation), sensation of fullness (bloating), increased formation of gas in abdomen, belching with bad taste in mouth, Kapha diseases of the stomach according to the Indian healing art of Ayurveda; feeling of heaviness in musculature, diseases of the mammary gland (mastopathy)

---

* In this case, speech disorders do not include stuttering.

Sector Li
Probability of illness: B
Gender: Female
Age: 48 to 65 years
Health Disorders: Feeling of heaviness in musculature

Sector Qian
Probability of illness: C
Gender: Female
Age: 65 and up
Health Disorders: Bone diseases (for example, osteoporosis, including the related tendency toward bone fractures)

Sector Dui
Probability of illness: C
Gender: Female
Age: 65 and up
Health Disorders: Adult-onset diabetes

Sector Sun
Probability of illness: D
Gender: Female
Age: 48 to 65 years
Health Disorders: Shen disorders (lack of drive, fatigue), lowered resistance, splenic enlargement

Trigram Dui (Birth Month Cock)

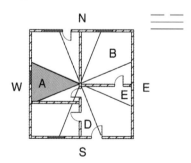

Sector Dui
Probability of illness: A
Gender: Female
Age: 0 to 16 years
Health Disorders: Saccharomycosis of oral cavity (thrush), teeth (defective jaw position), tooth spasms

Sector Gen
Probability of illness: B
Gender: Female
Age: 0 to 16 years
Health Disorders: Chronic swelling of nasal mucous membrane, disorders of sense of smell

Sector Li
Probability of illness: D
Gender: Female
Age: 0 to 16 years
Health Disorders: Acne, skin impurities

Sector Zhen
Probability of illness: E
Gender: Female
Age: Related to unborn who would have had their time of birth in a Dui month
Health Disorders: Female premature births

Trigram Qian (Birth Month Monkey)

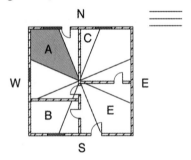

Sector Qian
Probability of illness: A
Gender: Male
Age: 48 to 65 years
Health Disorders: Diseases in head area* (frontal sinuses, ethmoidal cells, maxillary sinuses), headaches, cerebral arteriosclerosis**, respiratory diseases (bronchitis, chronic bronchitis), heart diseases*** (coronary arteriosclerosis)

---

* Health disorders in the head area include, for example, chronic mucous membrane swelling of the entire paranasal sinuses and their precursors, but tend less often to be acute inflammations. (Continued on pg. 193)

Sector Kun
Probability of illness: B
Gender: Male
Age: 48 to 65 years
Health Disorders: Degenerative nerve disease of the brain, spinal marrow, and the peripheral nerves (such as symmetrical polyneupathy), infertility (fertility disorder) through a disorder of the Jing

Sector Kan
Probability of illness: C
Gender: Male
Age: 65 and up
Health Disorders: Diseases of the bone marrow, nail diseases

Sector Sun
Probability of illness: E
Gender: Male
Age: 32 to 48 years
Health Disorders: Rubefaction (reddening of the skin), skin impurities

---

** Cerebral arteriosclerosis generally means the degenerative process of the cerebral arteries and/or its precursors, but not the phenomenon of acute strokes.

*** Heart diseases generally means the degenerative process of coronary sclerosis and/or its precursors, but not acute cardiac infarction.

Examples for a Person Who Has the Trigram Qian Above His or Her Birth Month (Monkey)

You see the trigram Qian in the list. Here you will find four possibly problematic sectors. So you must ask the four following questions:

"On the basis of my birth month, am I predispositioned to trigram-related health disorders when I sleep in the Qian sector?"

"On the basis of my birth month, am I predispositioned to trigram-related health disorders when I sleep in the Kun sector?"

"On the basis of my birth month, am I predispositioned to trigram-related health disorders when I sleep in the Kan sector?"

"On the basis of my birth month, am I predispositioned to trigram-related health disorders when I sleep in the Sun sector?"

The sectors **Zhen, Dui, Gen,** and **Li** do not cause problems here.

An Infant Drinks Properly Again

*Little Oliver's mother was practically in despair. After breast-feeding, he routinely vomited his food. It turned out that Oliver slept with his personal **trigram Gen** in the **sector Gen** of the house. The child's room was therefore moved. Two weeks later, the vomiting had stopped.*

Too Much Cholesterol in Sector Sun

*The 38-year-old Cornelia K. was not overweight, yet still had elevated cholesterol and neutral lipid values in her blood. She complained about pressure in the right upper abdomen after eating fatty foods, but no cause could be found by orthodox medicine. Ms. K. had the personal **trigram Sun** and slept in the **sector Sun** of the house. The locations of the bedroom and study were exchanged. After about eight weeks, the complaints in the upper abdomen area improved. The blood lipid values normalized as well.*

Menopause Complaints Improve

*A 45-year-old businesswoman was prematurely suffering from menopausal complaints with hot flashes and irregular menstruation with complaints in the lower abdomen. She had the personal **trigram Li** and slept in the **sector Kun**. The sleeping area was moved. The complaints improved after eight weeks.*

Problematic Trigram Sectors (Overview)

The following table gives you a summarized overview of the possible problem sectors, together with the probability of illness for the personal trigram of your birth month:

		Personal Trigram							
		Kan	Gen	Zhen	Sun	Li	Kun	Dui	Qian
Sector	Kan	A	E	B					C
	Gen	D	A	E				B	
	Zhen		D	A		B		E	
	Sun	C			A	B	D		E
	Li	E			C	A	B	D	
	Kun			E		C	A		B
	Dui			D		E	C	A	
	Qian				D	E	C		A

Aids

If you determine that a certain sector of the house is problematic for you as a sleeping area, it is best to use a Feng Shui Power Disc 99 or avoid that sector. However, it is frequently difficult to move the bedroom somewhere else. But even in you want to continue to sleep in the problematic sector without using a Feng Shui Power Disc 99, there are possibilities of at least diminishing the disruptive influence with the help of the **transformational materials** discussed in Chapter 7 on page 165 ff.

Which Transformational Materials in Which Sector?

If you have a problem in one sector of the house, consult the following table for the transformational materials you should use:

Sector	Transformational Materials (Number in parentheses shows life span of transformational materials in years)*
Kan	Wood: Wood (40), living plants (as long as they are alive), wood parquet (40), cork parquet (40), wicker baskets (5-7), drapes or floor covering of cotton or other plant fibers (2), chipboard (2), dried plants and ornamental gourds (1), books and magazines (1) (a place to store current magazines, which are replaced on a regular basis, would also be suitable for a longer period of time).
Gen	Metal: Gold bars (120), gold rings (80-90), steel (25-50), iron (40), brass (35), lead (25), aluminum (14), mercury (for example, in thermometers) (12), copper (11), tin (11), bronze (10), mirror coating (9), silver (6-10).
Zhen	Fire: Pebbles (practically unlimited), sheet glass (20-45), sheet glass in mirrors (20), candle flames and open fireplace fires (as long as they burn).
Sun	Fire: As described above.
Li	Earth: Crystals and gemstones (unlimited), natural stones (practically unlimited), porcelain (80-110), bricks (80), leather and furs (50-60), ceramics (50), concrete (30), wool carpets and other wool textiles (30), synthetics (20-25)**, natural silk (10-20), stearin candles (2), beeswax (1).
Kun	Metal: As described above.
Dui	Water: Blown glass (20), water.
Qian	Water: As above.

---

* This means that wood (40), for example, no longer can be used for the given purpose after approx. 40 years; brass (35) means that a brass object is also no longer useful for this purpose approx. 35 years after its manufacture (metal casting)

** Synthetically coated furniture on the basis of chipboard is solely the transformational material of earth after an age of about two years.

Gold Jewelry On the Nightstand in Sector Kun

Despite all kinds of diets, a 55-year-old woman complained about feeling bloated and experiencing increased gas formation in her abdomen. She had the month trigram of Kun. Up to now, she had kept her gold jewelry locked in a safe at night for security reasons. The feng shui consultant advised her to lay her gold jewelry on the nightstand next to the bed at night. Eight weeks later, her stomach complaints had improved to the point where she no longer had to adhere to any special diets.

A Glass Carafe with Water in the Sector Dui

A little girl was receiving medical treatment because of constantly recurring saccharomycosis in the oral cavity (thrush). In addition, she had already suffered three tooth spasms. She had the monthly trigram of Dui. At the advice of a feng shui consultant, the mother placed a glass carafe with fresh water next to the little girl's bed. The saccharomycosis of the oral cavity disappeared after two weeks. The mother also reported that there were no further tooth spasms.

Porcelain in the Bedroom in Sector Li

A 25-year-old woman had complained for years about circulatory problems with low blood pressure. Although she took cardiovascular drugs on a regular basis, she did not feel well. It turned out that the young woman with the month trigram of Li slept in the Li sector of the house. She was therefore advised to move the collection of Dresden china that stood in the dining room into her bedroom. Since she had enough room in the bedroom, she placed the china on a side table about one meter away from the bed. Four weeks later, her circulatory complaints had improved so much that she rarely had to take any cardiovascular drugs.

A Pine Bedroom Set in Sector Kan

A 43-year-old workman had a mycosis of a nail that was resistant to therapy. He had the month trigram of Zhen and slept in the Kan sector of the house. At this time, the bedroom furniture was made of synthetically coated chipboard. He had planned to buy new bedroom furniture within the next two years. He was advised to arrange for an earlier purchase date and select solid-wood furniture. He bought a complete new bedroom set made of solid pine wood. After 13 weeks, his complaints with the mycosis of the nail had disappeared.

Pebbles in Sector Zhen

A mother called a feng shui consultant because her eight-year-old son had been constantly having colds for the past two years. The boy had the month trigram of Gen. At the consultation, they discovered that the boy slept in the Zhen sector of the single-family home, in addition to other feng shui problems. A row of pebbles was placed on the small cupboard next to his bed. The mother reported that his susceptibility to infections had clearly improved after eight weeks.

Ask About the Transformational Materials

As you can see in the above case examples, integrating the appropriate transformational material in the bedroom is not too difficult. However, it is necessary to ask using the tensor or pendulum to find out what objects or measures are adequate in each specific case. So, if you sleep in a problematic sector of your house, first ask whether the addition of a suitable transformational material will adequately reduce the disruptive influence. The question is: *"Will the addition of the transformational material ... (name of the transformational material) in the bedroom be sufficient to compensate for the disruptive influence in the ... (sector name) sector?"* If you receive a YES, it is also necessary to find the appropriate object and the suitable place for it.

If you require the transformational material of wood in the Kan section, you can ask, for example: *"Is pine furniture made of solid wood suitable as a transformational material for compensating for the disruptive influence in the Kan sector?"*

If you receive a NO, ask about additional objects. When you receive a YES, continue to ask questions: *"Is it enough to place pine furniture of solid wood in this bedroom in order to balance out the disruptive influence in the Kan sector?"*

If you receive a YES, you have found the suitable object. If you receive a NO, ask about additional objects made of the transformational material of wood. It is frequently necessary to place a number of objects in the bedroom. Think about which objects could be suitable for this purpose.

Transformational materials should be placed as close to the bed as possible. If this is not possible for reasons of space, ask whether the planned location is adequately close to the bed using the tensor or pendulum.

Projection of the Trigram Sectors onto the Floor Plan of the House

In the previous section on *The Eight Trigrams and Their Sectors* on page 176, you have seen how you can determine the central point of your house on the basis of the floor plan. The drawings with the problematic trigram sectors have shown the position of the sectors for square houses that are oriented toward the north. If the house is not square, the angle of the individual sectors, seen from the central point of the house, remains constant. The orientation of the trigram sectors toward the directions also remains the same (see *Overview* on page 195: *The Eight Trigrams and Their Sectors* in the previous section on page 176).

We have found it practical to use a transparent foil for projecting the trigram sectors onto the floor plan of the house. You can make a transparent foil with the trigram sectors yourself by copying *The Eight Trigram Sectors* in the appendix of this book on page 243 onto transparent foil (if necessary, enlarge to standard paper size). The geographic direction of north is usually indicated with an arrow on house floor plans. Extend this arrow with the help of a ruler. In addition, mark the center point of your house, as described at the end of Chapter 7 on page 165 ff. Using a geometric triangle (a special ruler available in stationery stores), draw a line through the center point line of the house parallel to the extended arrow for the geographic direction of north. (If your geometric triangle is too small, you may possibly have to draw one or more additional parallel lines so that you reach the center point line of the house. Then lay the transparent foil on the floor plan of your house, placing the broken line of the transparent foil onto the center point line that you have just drawn. Where the lines cross on the transparent foil is now directly on the center point of the house. If you want to work with the trigram sectors of your house floor plan more extensively, we recommend that you copy the house floor plan with the properly aligned transparent foil on top of it.

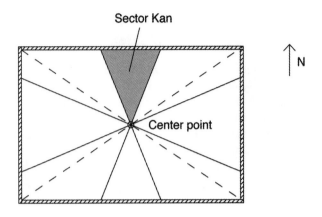

Projection of the trigram sectors onto a rectangular house that is oriented toward the north. The trigram sector Kan has been drawn in. The position of the other sectors results from the alignment of the main directions.

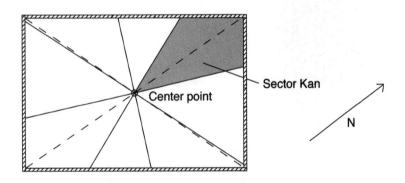

Projection of the trigram sectors onto a rectangular house that is not oriented toward the north. The trigram sector Kan has also been drawn in here.

When the Trigram Sectors Are Located Outside the House

The energies of feng shui require a house form in **the shape of a parallelepiped** for their complete development. Just having a rectangular or square floor plan alone is not enough. Instead, the entire spatial form of the house (including the cellar beneath it) is important for the distribution of the energies within the house.

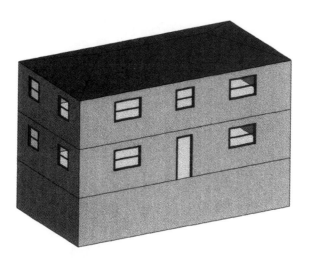

A parallelepiped-shaped house

If parts of the parallelepiped are excluded, a portion of the energies will be found outside the space that it has been built around. If a sector of the trigram lies in the area that has been left out in the house, this can have an effect similar to that of sleeping in this sector. However, this only applies when the sleeping area is located on the story whose floor plan shows an area that has been left out. If this left-out area, for example, is just on the top floor, but the sleep area is on the ground floor, this left-out area will not have an impact. The affected group of people can also be established on the basis of the birth month trigram. (You already know the trigram of your birth month.)

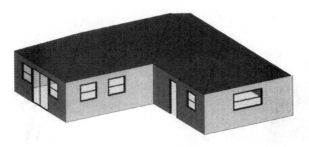

An L-shaped house

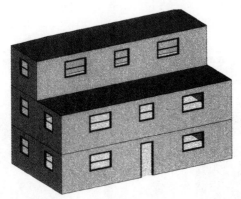

A house in which part of the upper floor has been left out.

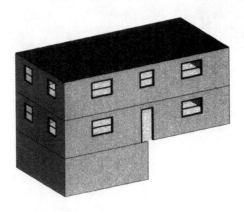

A house beneath only half of which there is a cellar. If a person sleeps in such a cellar (which can also cause problems for other feng shui reasons), on that floor it will be as if a part of the house is missing.

Predisposition Toward Health Disorders Because of Left-Out Areas of the House

It should be mentioned at this point again that the absorption of harmful energies by the human aura in the individual trigram sectors will be reduced to below the critical threshold with the Feng Shui Power Disc 99. This also applies to the problems in houses with left-out areas described here. If you live in an L-shaped house or in a house or on a story where a portion of it has been left out, you should once again clarify your personal predisposition with the tensor or pendulum if you have not placed a Feng Shui Power Disc 99 in the house. Independent of the fact that L-shaped houses or houses with recesses may have other feng shui problems because of their form, you can once again find the predisposition based on the trigram of your birth month, as described in the previous section on "The Eight Trigrams and Their Sectors." In this case, the left-out sectors or the left-out sectors of the floor plan of the story can be problematic. You must once again ask whether you actually have a predisposition toward illnesses here. While working through the previous section, you may have discovered that you can sleep in any sector of your house. However, you may have a problem if you sleep in a house or on a story with a left-out area that is located in a sector unfavorable for you.

With the help of the floor plan of your house, first clarify which sector or sectors are missing in your house or on the story where you sleep. At the end of the last section, you saw how you can project the trigram sectors (possibly with the help of a transparent foil) onto the floor plan of your house. The table on *Problematic Trigram Sectors* in the previous section on page 195 can help you discover what sectors are potentially problematic for you on the basis of the personal trigram of your birth month. If the left-out area in your house is not located in a sector that is problematic for you, then this area does not create any problems for you in terms of this approach. If trigram sectors are just partially missing, the influence is less than when they are completely or almost completely absent.

Ask About Your Predisposition Because of Left-Out Areas

You must therefore check: *"Because of my birth month, do I have a predisposition to trigram-related illnesses because the ... (sector name) sector is missing in my house?"*

Ask about the individual missing sectors and those that are problematic for you. If you receive a YES for a sector, read about the feng shui measures for it in the next section.

Example 1: If you have the personal trigram of the Qian birth month and the sectors Qian and Kan are missing in your house, ask the follow questions: *"Because of my birth month, do I have a predisposition to trigram-related illnesses because the Qian sector is missing in my house?"* and: *"Because of my birth month, do I have a predisposition to trigram-related illnesses because the Kan sector is missing in my house?"*

Example 2: You have the personal trigram of the Gen birth month and the sectors Kun and Dui are missing in your house, so you do not need to ask the above question because the sectors Kun and Dui are not problematic for a person with the trigram Gen in this respect.

You can also generally clarify your predisposition: *"Because of my birth month, do I have a predisposition to trigram-related illnesses when one or more sectors are missing in my house?"*

If you receive a NO, you can have your results checked by a second person who is also skilled and confident at working with the tensor or pendulum. The question would then be: *"Because of his/her birth month, does ... (name) generally have a predisposition to trigram-related illnesses when one or more sectors are missing in his/her house?"*

If this person also receives a NO, then you are not among the group of people who have this predisposition. You are then among the people who have no problems with these trigram aspects.

Feng Shui Measures for Left-Out Areas in the House

Even if you have already placed a Feng Shui Power Disc 99 in your house, it may be useful to also implement the feng shui remedies described here for other reasons. The goal of a feng shui measure is to extend an unfavorable floor plan or house form into a rectangle or parallelepiped. The **L-shape** is a house form frequently found in detached single-family houses. We recommend that you supplement this house form with something like a terrace to create a rectangle. This addition can be intensified by emphasizing the outside boundary of the terrace with a wall. Furthermore, it is beneficial to distinctly mark the outer edge of the terrace with a statue that looks toward the inside, a lantern, or in some other manner. Another possibility of complementing the form is planting a hedge to serve as the outer terrace boundary; the corner could be emphasized with a bush. There are similar supplementary possibilities for **U-shapes**, **cross shapes**, and **H-shapes**, as well as other non-rectangular forms. Semi-circles can be supplemented to form complete circles.

The **material** that you use to complete the imaginary rectangle should, if possible, consist of the same transformational material that you would use if you were sleeping in the problematic sector. We also recommend that you additionally place this transformational material in the trigram sector located outside the house. You can find the suitable transformational material in the table on *Which Transformational Materials in Which Sector* on page 195.

Nighttime Voiding Because of Missing Trigram Sector Kan

A 22-year-old woman had been having urological treatment for 1 1/2 years because of a nervous bladder. She had to get up about three times a night to urinate. Her mother therefore advised her to get advice from a feng shui consultant. During the consultation, it became clear that the trigram sector Kan was missing in the L-shaped house. The trigram of the young woman's birth month was also Kan. In addition to other measures, the feng shui consultant advised her to make the house into a rectangle by planting a green hedge and placing a bush in the corner of this imaginary rectangle. The hedge and bush were planted as recommended in the spring of the next year. Terrace furniture made of plastic was replaced by wooden furniture. Six months later, the young woman's complaints had improved to the point that she only had to get up once a night.

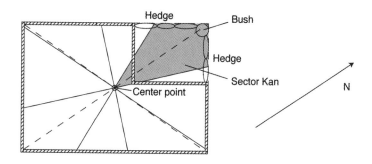

Because the trigram sector Kan was missing, an L-shaped house was extended into a rectangle by planting a hedge and a bush.

Muscle Cramps Because of Missing Trigram Sector Zhen

A 22-year-old woman had been complaining for more than three years about muscle spasms in her legs, particularly at night. She took mineral supplements on a regular basis, but the complaints flared up time and again. The young woman lived in an L-shaped house in which the eastern corner had been left out. So the trigram sector Zhen was missing. The trigram of the young woman's birth month was Li. The feng shui consultant recommended that the house form be extended into a rectangle by using the transformational material of fire. In the corner of the imaginary rectangle, they placed a copper can that was about 20 years old and filled it with pebbles. In addition, pebbles were strewn along the imaginary boundary. An old copper can that no longer functioned as the transformational material of metal was deliberately selected. Four months later, the woman reported that for the first time in years she had been able to get through the night without muscle spasms. (Because of other feng shui reasons, pebbles should not be used extensively as a material for the floor of a terrace.)

If the trigram sector **Li** is missing, it is possible to place a statue in the imaginary corner of the rectangle and to additionally build a natural stone wall on the imaginary line; a stone bank could also be installed.

If the trigram sector **Kun** is missing, it would be possible to place a metal statue in the imaginary corner of the rectangle. However, when you place additional metal in the trigram sector Kun, be sure that no Trans-Sha gets into the house as a result.

If the trigram sector **Dui** is missing, place a glass bowl with fresh water or a small waterfall in the imaginary corner of the rectangle. A pond should not be built within the trigram sector. We also tend to advise against a fountain within the trigram sector. This should be placed close to the outside line of the plot of land that has been extended to form a rectangle.

Chapter 9

Animal-Sign Sectors and Health

The Animal-Sign Sectors

In Chapter 8 we discussed the meaning of the Chinese animal signs of the birth month in the section on *Trigram Sectors Can Influence Your Health* on page 180. This chapter is concerned with the meaning of the Chinese animal signs of the birth year.

The twelve Chinese animal signs are assigned respectively to two adjacent sectors of the inner aura structure of the house. This means that each animal-sign sector comprises 15 degrees and that there is always an empty 15 degree sector between two animal-sign sectors.

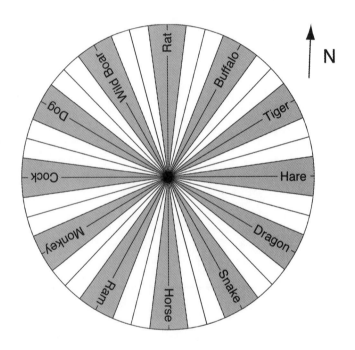

The twelve animal signs and their sectors (chart for copying in the appendix on page 240).

Chinese Animal Sign of Year	Yin/Yang Classification, Wu Xing	Direction*
Rat	Yang—Water	349.9-4.9 degrees
Buffalo (or Ox)	Yin—Earth	19.9-34.9 degrees
Tiger	Yang—Wood	49.9-64.9 degrees
Hare (or Rabbit)	Yin—Wood	79.9-94.9 degrees
Dragon	Yang—Earth	109.9-124.9 degrees
Snake	Yin—Fire	139.9-154.9 degrees
Horse	Yang—Fire	169.9-184.9 degrees
Ram (or Sheep)	Yin—Earth	199.9-214.9 degrees
Monkey	Yang—Metal	229.9-244.9 degrees
Cock	Yin—Metal	259.9-274.9 degrees
Dog	Yang—Earth	289.9-304.9 degrees
Wild Boar (or Pig)	Yin—Water	319.9-334.9 degrees

Disruptive Influences in the Sectors of the Animal Signs

Some people—or the simpler portions of these people's minds—react particularly sensitively to certain influences in the sector of the house to which their animal sign is assigned. These are influences that essentially have an effect on the simpler mental portions of a human through the aura. They are capable of perceiving disruptions in the sectors of the house's aura structures that are assigned to the animal sign of a person's birth year with particular intensity. In this process, they are distinctly receptive to disruptions at night. It is not necessary for the person to actually be present in the respective area. It is enough for the disruptive sector of the aura structure to be in the kinetic range of the mental portion. This kinetic area extends, as described, generally to the first hull of the house's outer aura.

---

* The stated number of degrees is related to the geographic direction of north.

The simpler mental portions have the task, among other things, of controlling a human being's bodily functions and correcting them, if necessary. They also have these tasks at night, although normally with less effort, because the body is asleep. However, if their attention is distracted by processes interesting them in one the sector of the house with which their animal sign is associated, it may happen that they transfer the mechanisms of these processes to the way in which the body functions. This can lead to health disorders. Fortunately, only about 12% of all human beings are potentially affected by this problem. It is therefore sensible to ask whether you even belong to this group by using the tensor or pendulum. If you have placed a Feng Shui Power Disc 99 in the house, this excessive interest of the simpler mental portions in the technical processes in their respective animal section will diminish.

Check to See Whether You Are Receptive to Influences from Your Animal-Sign Sector

Ask: *"On the basis of my birth year, am I receptive to influences from my animal-sign sector?"*

If you receive a NO, you can also have the results checked by a second person, who is skilled and confident at working with the tensor or pendulum. The question is then: *"On the basis of his/her birth year, is ... (name) receptive to influences from his/her animal-sign sector?"*

If this person also receives a NO, you are not among the group of potentially receptive people. So you do not need to take this aspect into consideration.

If you have received a YES, look for your animal-sign sector in your house if you haven't already placed a Feng Shui Power Disc 99 in your house. For this purpose, once again use a floor plan, as already described for the trigram sectors. For the animal-sign sectors as well, you can make a transparent foil with the help of the "12 Animal-Sign Sectors" chart to be copied in the appendix of the book (if necessary, enlarge to standard paper size). Place the transparent foil on the floor plan as already described for the trigram sectors. If you want to work with the animal-sign sectors of your house floor plan over a longer period of time, we again suggest that you copy the house floor plan together with the transparent foil placed on it and oriented correctly.

Within this context, the influences that are found on the story where your bedroom is also located are relevant. So if you sleep on the 2nd floor of your house, you only need to take into consideration the influences found on the 2nd floor of your house. However, pay attention that the central point of the house, from which the animal-sign sectors radiate, is related to the central point of the entire house. This is significant when the surface of the floor that you sleep on is smaller than the overall surface of the house.

What Can Have a Disruptive Effect in the Animal-Sign Sectors?

The individual animal signs are particularly receptive for the influences of objects and/or installations assigned to them in the following list. This means that if such an object or such an installation is found in the animal-sign sector of a potentially receptive person, there is a great probability that the influence actually has an effect. However, it is possible that objects or installations mentioned under the other animal signs can also have an effect.

Disruptive Influences in the Animal-Sign Sectors

Chinese Animal Sign of the Year	Frequently Found Disruptive Objects and Installations: Effect
Rat	• No specific influences
Buffalo (or Ox)	• Gas heating: lungs • House altars: excessive self-confidence
Tiger	• Vacuum cleaner: large intestine/diarrhea • Household steam cleaner: large intestine
Hare (or Rabbit)	• No specific influences
Dragon	• Eaves and gutters: lymph (rare) • Transmitting units: disturb the orientation
Snake	• Entrance and exit (for example, waste water) feeding pipes and lines into the house (main water pipe, electrical lines): not good for the teeth • Electrical bread-cutting machines and mixers: not good for the teeth • Chimney: ethmoidal cells

Horse	• Transmitting units: disturb the orientation
Ram (or Sheep)	• Waste-water tank: kidneys
	• Bathtub: kidneys
	• Shower: kidneys
	• Dishwasher: kidneys
	• Computer on the Internet: dissatisfaction
Monkey	• Bathtub: kidneys
	• Shower: kidneys
	• Freezer or freezer compartment of refrigerator: symptoms of cold
Cock	• Eaves and gutters: lymph
	• Fountains: tendency toward infections
Dog	• Answering machine: becoming too lazy to talk
	• CD player: weakens sense of orientation
	• Electrical bread-cutting machines and mixers: not good for teeth
	• Dishwasher: kidneys
Wild Boar (or Pig)	• CD player: weakens sense of orientation
	• Gas connection: veins
	• Computer on the Internet: dissatisfaction

Further Influence Possibilities

In individual cases, other objects and/or installations can also have a disruptive effect. We should at least mention **gas stoves and electrical ranges**, which can produce symptoms of heat; the gas stoves have a more intensive effect in this regard than electrical ranges. **Machines with a large motor** can also impede the functioning of the heart.

When people are potentially receptive, we recommend that you ask whether an influence is actually effective during the night. To do this, you should go to the respective animal-sign sector. There you should ask: *"Are there influences in this animal-sign sector that have an effect on me at night based on my birth year?"*

If you receive a NO, have your result checked by a second person. If this person also receives a NO, then you may belong to the group of potentially receptive people, but there are no objects and/or installations in your animal-sign sector at the moment that could influence you. Also, make sure that you do not place any of these objects or installations there in the future.

If you receive a YES, then look for the objects or installations with the question: *"Does ... (name of object or installation have an effect on me during the night on the basis of my birth year?"*

Ask about the individual objects and installations. Remember that there may be more than one object or installation causing a disturbance. To be sure, ask in closing: *"Have I found all the objects and/or installations that have an effect on me during the night on the basis of my birth year?"*

If you receive a NO, keep searching. If you receive a YES, there are a number of possibilities:

1) Place a Feng Shui Power Disc 99 in the house.
2) Remove the object and/or installation from your animal-sign sector.
3) Change your sleeping area to another story.
4) Since permanently installed furnishings can be especially problematic to move and a change of the sleeping place to another story is not always possible, it is necessary to distract the simpler portions of the human mind during the night in the respective animal-sign sector. This is possible when you find something that is more attractive to it than the disruptive object or the installation. The simpler portions of the human mind like to turn to certain fragrances, like those emanating from some types of fruit and plant juices. Next, it is a matter of finding the appropriate fruit or plant juices that are adequately effective.

Remedies for Disruptive Influences in the Animal-Sign Sectors

Chinese Animal Signs of the Year	*Suitable Fruit or Plant Juices*
Rat	Apple juice (sour, naturally cloudy), elder-blossom juice, cherry juice (not sour but sweet cherries)
Buffalo (or Ox)	Red grape juice, red cabbage juice, sorrel juice, sugar-beet juice

Tiger	Carrot juice (best with honey, not lemon), beet juice, tomato juice
Hare (or Rabbit)	White grape juice
Dragon	Sauerkraut juice, elder-blossom juice, elder-berry juice, stinging-nettle juice, mistletoe juice
Snake	Lemon juice, red-cabbage juice
Horse	Peach juice, hawthorn juice
Ram (or Sheep)	Orange juice, grapefruit juice, stinging-nettle juice
Monkey	Apricot juice, birch juice
Cock	Cherry juice (not sour but sweet cherry), radish juice
Dog	Orange, lemon, lime, tangerine, blood-orange, and citrus juices (except grapefruit)
Wild Boar (or Pig)	Blueberry juice, red-pepper juice

Two drops of juice placed in the respective animal-sign sector during the night are enough. Take a little bowl (diameter of 2 1/2 inches or 6 centimeters) filled with water and add two drops of juice to it. The water with the juice must be replaced every three days. It is generally adequate to carry out this procedure for about eight weeks. After about eight weeks, use the tensor or pendulum to ask whether the effect was adequate. If you receive a NO, continue placing the water and the juice in the sector for two more weeks. If you receive a YES, it is generally necessary to repeat this procedure after one year has passed. At that time, once again place the water with the two drops of juice in the sector for about eight weeks. It is usually not necessary to repeat the process for more than six years.

Another possibility is to use plant juices of cold-soaked leaf or plant extracts of the above-named plants. The leaves or plants should soak in cold water for two days. The extract is then ready and can be poured through a sieve. Use the extract without diluting it and also renew it after three days.

Outlook

You have learned some things about examining and clearing up the sleeping area in this book. We have attempted to integrate everything essential for your health. If you follow our advice, you will lay a good foundation for maintaining or even improving your health and your well-being at home.

What other possibilities does the system of feng shui offer in addition to what you have learned here?

The Proper Place for a House

The system of feng shui can help you in selecting the proper, as well as "auspicious," place for your house. This not only applies to your private home, but also to various types of business buildings. The proper choice of your living and working rooms is often the first step in creating a place for your ideas and translating them into reality. Harmony, in both the private and the business sense, can only properly develop when you activate the energies and forces of the right place.

The Invisible Inner Life of the House

We have already given you an insight into the inner aura structure of the house. Beyond the health considerations, the system of feng shui will give you the possibility of designing the interior of your house in such a way that both the happiness of your family and success in your working life are intensified. The Chinese have long been concerned with keeping "evil spirits" and outside energies away from their homes. They have been particularly interested in protecting the house from outside influences.

Feng Shui—The Compass School

You already received a small insight into the Compass School of feng shui when we introduced the trigram sectors and the animal-sign sectors, as well as their meaning for your health. To a large extent, the direction that the house faces determines the distribution of the energies in the house. Important influences are the time of the house's completion, the occupant's time of birth, and current time influences of the year, month, day, and the Chinese double hour.

Feng Shui of Time

The choice of the right point in time plays a large role in implementing a project. On the basis of the "Four Pillars of Destiny" (Ba Zi Suan), you can determine at which point in time a certain project is auspicious for a person. If the time is unfavorable, it is often better to postpone the activities for a while. Only the combination of the right point in time with the right place brings feng shui's possibilities to full blossom.

Appendix

Glossary

Acceleration

In order for an energy from a higher dimension to pass into a lower dimension, it must be accelerated. Energies that are accelerated from the 5th or 4th dimension into our own (3rd) dimension are important for us.

Analytical School

In the Analytical School of feng shui, influences that have an effect on a human being in a specific place and at a certain time are directly perceived. In order to determine these influences, the Analytical School uses the L-rod, tensor, or pendulum.

Animal Signs

The Chinese assign the twelve Chinese animal signs to both the years and months. These should not be confused with the twelve Western signs of the Zodiac. The Chinese animal signs are: Rat, Buffalo, Tiger, Hare, Dragon, Snake, Horse, Ram, Monkey, Cock, Dog, and Wild Boar.

Aura

Aura is the term used for the subtle bodies of a human being and for the subtle structure within a house and surrounding a house.

Cellular Glass Plates of a Suitable Quality

Particularly in the construction of a house, cellular glass plates can be used as shielding material against harmful energies in the sleeping area and at the workplace. It is important to know that the qualities usually available often do not create the desired effect.

Chemical Effects, Negative

A negative impact on the health of the occupants of a house can occur particularly because of solvents, wood preservatives, and heavy metals.

Clock Radios with Red Digital Display

Clock radios with red digital displays (above all, cheap products from the Far East) activate Per-Sha when the red numbers are illuminated. This has a negative effect similar to that of Geo-Sha.

Compass School

In the plains of Northern China, an extensive system for evaluating a place on the basis of the influences from the directions, as well as on temporal factors, was developed. The evaluation of energies is done with the help of the feng shui compass (Luopan).

Cork of a Suitable Quality

Cork tiles and cork parquet can be used particularly for correcting sleeping environments since they form a protective structure. It is important to know that the qualities usually available generally do not create the desired effect.

Direction-Dependent Cube System

A direction-dependent cube system is a structure in the earth's magnetic field, used for the conveyance of energies. It cannot be proved with physical methods of measurement. However, it is possible to find it using the L-rod, tensor, or pendulum. In particular, the side walls of certain cube systems should be avoided during sleep. We describe the Hartmann System, as well as the 10-Meter, 170-Meter, and 250-Meter System, in this book. In the side walls of the 10-Meter and 250-Meter System, Geo-Sha is conducted downward. In the side walls of the 170-Meter and Hartmann System, Trans-Sha is conducted upward. Furthermore, the side walls of the Hartmann System conduct Per-Sha upward in the vicinity of fault zones.

Dimension

In the system of feng shui, there are 7 dimensions. We live in the 3rd dimension.

Divining

Another term for finding invisible structures and energies using the dowsing rod, tensor, pendulum, or L-rod.

Electrosmog

Electromagnetic influences of various types are summarized by this term.

Energy, Intensity of

Not only the type of energy, but also the intensity of energy can be determined with the tensor or pendulum. There are two possible ways of stating the intensity of an energy:

A) We determine the intensity of an energy on a scale from 0 to 100.

B) We determine whether the intensity of an energy is above or below a person's individual threshold value.

Fault Zones

Faults in the crust of the earth activate two harmful types of Per-Sha, which in this case rise upward in a slightly fan-shaped form. These energies have a yang effect on human beings.

Feng Shui Power Disc 99

The Feng Shui Power Disc 99 protects the house against harmful energies (Geo-Sha, Trans-Sha, and Per-Sha), increases beneficial energies (Vital-Qi, Perm-Qi), and simultaneously has a good effect on a large number of other feng shui problems in the house.

Feng Shui Remedies for Correction and Vitalization

There is a possibility of reducing the harmful energies (Geo-Sha, Trans-Sha, and Per-Sha, if present) in the house while simultaneously increasing the beneficial energies (Vital-Qi, Perm-Qi). Examples of these are the Feng Shui Power Disc 99 and silica discs.

Form School

In the mountainous regions of Southern China, the so-called Form School of feng shui was developed. By observing the forms of the landscape and rivers, a differentiated valuation of the individual forms was developed in terms of their positive and negative effects on human beings.

Geo-Sha

Geo-Sha is an energy harmful to human beings and can be found in the side walls of certain geomagnetic cube systems. Geo-Sha moves in a downward direction. The harmful effect on human beings is most intense during sleep.

Hartmann Cube System

The Hartmann Cube System is abbreviated as the Hartmann System. In the vicinity of watercourses, it conducts Trans-Sha upward in its side walls. In the vicinity of fault zones, it conducts Per-Sha upward in its side walls.

Individual Need

The individual need for a positive energy indicates how much a specific person requires of this energy. In this process, the tensor or pendulum determines whether the individual need for this energy is covered or not.

Individual Threshold

The individual threshold for a harmful energy indicates how much a specific person tolerates on a scale of 0 to a maximum of 100 without becoming ill. The individual threshold value for Geo-Sha, Trans-Sha, and Per-Sha is usually between 4 and 5.

Intersection Points

The passing of energies between the dimensions takes place at the so-called intersection points. These invisible intersection points assume the form of a lens or spiral. Intersection points are often found in the side walls of geomagnetic cube systems.

Level

The invisible world has 32 levels. Of these, we call 10 levels subtle. The other 22 levels we call non-materil.l. Levels does not mean planes in space but rather the various degrees of subtleness.

Li

The Chinese call all types of structures Li.

Life Span of Feng Shui Remedies that Correct and Vitalize

The life span of the Feng Shui Power Disc 99 is about 50 years. The life span for the silica discs when used for the purposes described here is about 8 years. This only applies when these materials for feng shui remedies are not damaged.

Life Span of Materials that Create a Protective Structure

The effective life varies in length. For cellular glass plates of a suitable quality, it is 60 years; for cork of a suitable quality, it is 40 years; for XEPS plates it is 8 to 9 years.

Life Span of Transformational Materials

The effective life of so-called transformational materials is limited. This means that these materials are no longer capable of activating the Laws of Change after a specific period of time.

L-Rod

The L-shaped rod (L-shaped dowsing rod, also abbreviated to L-rod) is especially used to find subtle structures. In general, people work with two L-rods at the same time. The short arm of the L-rod is held by the hand so that the long arm above the hand points forward in a somewhat horizontal direction. If there is a YES reaction, the long arms turn toward each other. If there is a NO reaction, the long arms turn outward.

Metals

When metals are placed in the side walls of geomagnetic cube systems or above watercourses, they activate Trans-Sha and lead to a loss of Vital-Qi in the room.

Mirrors

Because of their metal portions, mirrors frequently create problems with Trans-Sha. For a number of different reasons, they do not belong in the bedroom.

Moon Stripes

Moon stripes are part of the inner structure of a direction-dependent cube system. They can have an unfavorable effect on human beings through Geo-Sha or trigger a certain type of restlessness.

Pendulum

With the pendulum, you can determine the type and intensity of energies and look for subtle structures. It makes it possible for you to receive answers in the form of YES and NO to questions of various types.

Perm-Qi

Perm-Qi is a positive energy for human beings. It is a type of Qi.

Per-Sha

Per-Sha is the name we give to the various energies that have a diagonal direction of flow in the 5th dimension. We find these energies above fault zones and in clock radios with red digital displays and satellite dishes. They have an unfavorable effect on human beings.

Polyxans

Polyxans are homeopathic potency accords of "carex flava." They are used to reduce the negative impact of Geo-Sha, Trans-Sha, and Per-Sha.

Qi (Spoken chee)

The Chinese frequently summarize the energies that are positive for human beings under the term of Qi. Since the various positive energies behave in different ways, we have used the terms Perm-Qi, Vital-Qi, and Shen in this book. The Japanese use the same character for the term as the Chinese, but pronounce it as Ki (as in Reiki).

Sector

The inner structure of a house's aura consists of 48 equally large sectors. A number of these sectors are summarized as the so-called trigram sectors and the animal-sign sectors, among other things.

Sha

The Chinese use the general term of Sha to summarize the energies that are negative for human beings. In this book, we have given the individual harmful energies various names (see *Geo-Sha, Trans-Sha,* and *Per-Sha* on page 49 ff).

Shen

The Chinese use the term Shen for positive energies, particularly those that have an effect on the human mind.

Tensor

The tensor is the modern form of the dowser. It is held with one hand. You can determine the type and intensity of energies and look for subtle structures with the tensor. The tensor makes it possible for you to receive answers to various types of questions in the form of YES and NO.

Transformational Materials

Transformational Materials are materials that activate the Five Laws of Change (Wu Xing).

Trans-Sha

Trans-Sha is the term we use for an energy that has a horizontal direction of flow in the 5th dimension. When this energy comes into our dimension, it has an inauspicious effect on human beings. We find Trans-Sha coming from below into the side walls of certain geomagnetic cube systems and above swirling water. Trans-Sha that has been activated by inauspiciously placed metals also tends to have a horizontal path in our dimension. Its degree of harmfulness is approximately the same as that of Geo-Sha.

Trigram

A trigram consists of a combination of three horizontal lines. The solid line represents yang, and the broken line represents yin. The eight trigrams are called: Kan, Gen, Zhen, Sun, Li, Kun, Dui, and Qian.

Vital-Qi

Vital-Qi is an energy that is positive for human beings. It is a type of Qi.

Watercourses

A watercourse with swirling water activates the so-called Trans-Sha that comes from below and rises upward, which is harmful for human beings.

WS Frequency Device

The WS Frequency Device is employed for reducing the negative effect of Geo-Sha, Trans-Sha, and Per-Sha. WS stands for "wide spectrum." The device is based on the healing effect of a selected natural stone powder, which is applied to ceramic rods and heated. It can also be used for a great variety of healing purposes.

Wu Xing

Wu Xing can be translated as the "Five Laws of Change." The Five Laws of Change lead to certain energy qualities in our dimension. These have the names of: Wood, Fire, Earth, Metal, and Water. The translation of "Five Elements" is occasionally found, but this translation is actually misleading.

XEPS Plates

The extruded polystyrene hard foam plates form a protective structure against harmful energies in the sleeping area and at the workplace. The following brand names are suitable for feng shui purposes: Styrofoam High Load 40, Styrofoam High Load 60, and Styrofoam High Load 100 from the Dow Chemical Company.

Yin and Yang

Yin and yang describe two opposite aspects of the same thing. So the human being is feminine and masculine. The front side of the human being is yin, and the back side is yang; the left side is yin, the right side is yang; the lower portion is yin, the upper portion is yang; and so forth.

Instructions for Constructing the Tensor and Pendulum

There are brief instructions for constructing a pair of L-rods under *You Can Measure Subtle Structures with the L-Rod* on page 22.

A) Tensor

We need three things in order to build a tensor:

1) Handle
2) Flexible wire
3) Weight on the tip

On 1)

The handle can be made of wood, metal, plastic, or some other material. It must fit well into your hand. The length of the handle should be 4–6 inches (10–15 cm). The diameter depends upon the material. The diameter of a metal handle should be about 3/8 inches (10 mm); 6/8 to 9/8 inches (20–30 mm) have proved to be effective for lighter materials like wood or plastic.

On 2)

The flexible wire consists of a steel wire with a diameter of about 1/16 inch (1 mm). The free length of the wire between the handle and the weight at the tip is about 12 inches (30 cm).

On 3)

A ring or ball have proved to be effective as the weight at the tip. Common models with a ring have rings in the form of a flat disk with an outside diameter of about 11/8 inches (34 mm) and an inside diameter of about 7/8 inches (22 mm) with a height just over 1/16 inch (about 2 mm).

There are also rod models made completely of plastic, whereby the distance to the weight at the tip is usually greater than 12 inches (30 cm).

B) Pendulum

A pendulum consists of:
1) A pendulum head
2) A pendulum cord

On 1)

The pendulum head is normally a cone, the tip of which points downward. However, you can also use another object with a weight of approx. 12 to 50 grams. Even a ring (like a wedding ring) is suitable as the head of a pendulum.

On 2)

The pendulum cord can be a normal string, a cord, or chain. The pendulum head is attached to the lower end of the pendulum cord, and you hold the upper part of the pendulum cord between your thumb and index finger or between the index and middle finger, depending on what feels best to you. The distance between the pendulum head and the hand should be about 4 to 6 inches (10 to 15 cm). The optimal distance is dependent upon the weight of the pendulum head and the type of purpose the pendulum is meant to serve. Experiment to find the best distance for you.

The Chinese Lunar Calendar

Here are examples of looking for the Chinese animal sign of the year and the month and a given date of birth (the times are based on Greenwich Mean Time/GMT; there is information on translating the time to your own time zone at the end of this section):

1) Date of birth: July 16, 1924

In the line next to the number of the year 1924, you will find the animal sign of the Rat. The corresponding Chinese lunar year begins on 2/05/1924 at 1:38am GMT and ends on 1/24/1925 at 2:45pm GMT. There is no doubt that 7/16/1924 belongs to the animal sign of the *Year of the Rat.*

The Chinese lunar month for the given date is the 6th month with the *Ram as the animal sign of the month.* This month begins on 7/02/1924 at 5:35am GMT and ends on 7/31/1924 at 7:42pm GMT. The personal trigram is then GEN for women and KUN for men.

2) Date of birth: January 12, 1957

The corresponding *animal sign of the year* is *Monkey.* Notice that the Chinese lunar year stated in the line next to 1956 extends from 2/11/1956 at 9:38pm GMT to 1/30/1957 at 9:25pm GMT. The Chinese lunar year and the year calculated in Western terms are not exactly alike.

The *animal sign of the month* is *Buffalo.* The corresponding Chinese lunar month begins on 1/1/1957 at 2:14pm GMT and ends on 1/30/1957 at 9:25pm GMT. The beginning on 1/1 is purely coincidental and has nothing to do with the new year according to the Western calendar. The personal trigram is GEN.

3) Date of birth: January 28, 1960 at 11am GMT

The *animal sign of the year* is *Rat.* The corresponding year begins on 1/28/1960 at 6:15pm GMT and ends on 2/15/1952 at 12:10am GMT.

The *animal sign of the month* is *Tiger.* The corresponding Chinese lunar month begins on 1/28/1960 at 6:15pm GMT and ends on 2/26/1960 at 6:24pm GMT. The personal trigram is ZHEN.

4) Date of birth: June 2, 1982

The *animal sign of the year* is **Dog**. The *animal sign of the month* is **Snake**. We find the date of 4/23 in the calendar marked with a star:*. This means that a lunar month begins on 4/23 that follows a so-called "leap" month. Leap months are necessary since the Chinese lunar calendar is just a little longer than 29.5 days. Since leap months are assigned to the same Chinese animal sign as the previous month, their beginning dates are not listed separately. The corresponding lunar month with the animal sign of snake therefore begins on 4/23/1982 at 8:29pm GMT. The following leap month ends on 6/21/1982 at 11:52am GMT. The personal trigram is LI.

Note:

If you were born during the transition from one month to another, your birth time must be translated into GMT. Also make allowances for possible shifts caused by Daylight Savings Time in the time zone of your birth. If you have difficulty with this calculation, a (Western) astrologer can help you. Exact details of the time zones taking into account the Daylight Savings Time of past (as well as future) years for various cities in the USA can also be found in: Thomas G. Shanks, *The American Atlas*, ACS Publications. For information on cities in other countries, consult: Thomas G. Shanks, *The International Atlas*, ACS Publications.

Lunar Calendar 1900–1919

(Greenwich Mean Time/GMT)

		1st Tiger	2nd Hare	3rd Dragon	4th Snake	5th Horse
1900	*Rat*	1/31 1:23am	3/1 11:25am	3/30 8:30pm	4/29 5:23am	5/28 2:50pm
1901	*Buffalo*	2/19 2:45am	3/20 12:53pm	4/18 9:37pm	5/18 4:38am	6/16 1:33pm
1902	*Tiger*	2/8 1:21pm	3/10 2:50am	4/8 1:50pm	5/7 10:45pm	6/6 6:11am
1903	*Hare*	1/28 4:38pm	2/27 10:19am	3/29 1:26am	4/27 1:31pm	5/26* 10:50pm
1904	*Dragon*	2/16 11:05am	3/17 5:39am	4/15 9:53pm	5/15 10:58am	6/13 9:10pm
1905	*Snake*	2/4 11:06am	3/6 5:19am	4/5 11:23pm	5/4 3:50pm	6/3 5:56am
1906	*Horse*	1/24 5:09pm	2/23 7:57am	3/24 11:52pm	4/23* 4:06pm	6/21 11:05pm
1907	*Ram*	2/12 5:43pm	3/14 6:05am	4/12 8:06pm	5/12 8:59am	6/10 11:50pm
1908	*Monkey*	2/2 8:36am	3/2 6:57pm	4/1 5:02am	4/30 3:33pm	5/30 3:14am
1909	*Cock*	1/22 11:12am	2/20* 10:52am	4/20 4:51am	5/19 1:42pm	6/17 11:28pm
1910	*Dog*	2/10 1:13am	3/11 12:12pm	4/9 9:25pm	5/9 5:33am	6/7 1:16pm
1911	*Wild Boar*	1/30 9:44am	3/1 12:31am	3/30 12:38pm	4/28 10:25pm	5/28 8:24am
1912	*Rat*	2/18 5:44am	3/18 10:08pm	4/17 11:40am	5/16 10:13pm	6/15 6:23am
1913	*Buffalo*	2/6 5:22am	3/8 12:22am	4/6 5:48pm	5/6 8:24am	6/4 7:57pm
1914	*Tiger*	1/26 7:34am	2/25 1:02am	3/26 7:09pm	4/25 12:21pm	5/26* 3:34am
1915	*Hare*	2/14 5:31	3/15 8:42pm	4/14 12:35pm	5/14 4:31am	6/12 7:57pm
1916	*Dragon*	2/3 4:05pm	3/4 3:57pm	4/2 4:21pm	5/2 5:29am	5/31 7:37pm
1917	*Snake*	1/23 7:40am	2/21 6:09pm	3/23* 4:05am	5/21 12:46am	6/19 1:02pm
1918	*Horse*	2/11 10:04am	3/12 7:52pm	4/11 4:34am	5/10 1:01pm	6/8 :02pm
1919	*Ram*	1/31 11:07pm	3/2 11:11am	3/31 9:04pm	4/30 5:30am	5/29 1:12pm

6th Ram	7th Monkey	8th Cock	9th Dog	10th Wild Boar	11th Rat	12th Buffalo
6/27 1:27am	7/26 1:43pm	8/25* 3:53am	10/23 1:27pm	11/22 7:17am	12/22 12:01am	1/20/01 2:36pm
7/15 10:10pm	8/14 8:27am	9/12 9:19pm	10/12 1:11pm	11/11 7:34am	12/11 2:53am	1/9/02 9:14pm
7/5 12:59pm	8/3 8:17pm	9/2 5:19am	10/1 5:09pm	10/31 8:14am	11/30 2:04am	12/29 9:25pm
7/24 12:46pm	8/22 7:51pm	9/21 4:31am	10/20 3:30pm	11/19 5:10am	12/18 9:26pm	1/17/04 3:47pm
7/13 5:27am	8/11 12:58pm	9/9 8:43pm	10/9 5:25am	11/7 3:37pm	12/7 3:46am	1/5/15 6:17pm
7/2 5:50pm	8/1 4:02am	8/30 1:13pm	9/28 9:59pm	10/28 6:58am	11/26 4:47pm	12/26 4:04am
7/21 12:59pm	8/20 1:27am	9/18 12:33pm	10/17 10:43pm	11/16 10:43pm	12/15 6:54pm	1/14/07 5:57am
7/10 3:17pm	8/9 6:36am	9/7 9:04pm	10/7 10:20am	11/5 10:39pm	12/5 10:22am	1/3/08 9:43pm
6/28 4:31pm	7/28 7:17am	8/26 10:59pm	9/25 2:39pm	10/25 6:46am	11/23 9:53pm	12/22 11:50am
7/17 10:45am	8/15 11:54pm	9/14 3:08pm	10/14 8:13am	11/13 2:18am	12/12 7:58pm	1/10/10 11:51am
7/6 9:20pm	8/5 6:37am	9/3 6:06pm	10/3 8:32am	11/2 1:56am	12/1 9:10pm	12/31 4:21pm
6/26* 1:19pm	8/24 4:14am	9/22 2:37pm	10/22 4:09am	11/20 8:49pm	12/20 3:40pm	1/19/12 11:10am
7/14 1:13pm	8/12 7:57pm	9/11 3:48am	10/10 1:40pm	11/9 2:05am	12/8 5:06pm	1/07/13 10:28am
7/4 5:06am	8/2 12:58pm	8/31 8:38pm	9/30 4:57am	10/29 2:29pm	11/28 1:41am	12/27 2:58pm
7/23 2:38am	8/21 12:26pm	9/19 9:33pm	10/19 6:33am	11/17 4:02pm	12/17 2:35am	1/15/15 2:43pm
7/12 9:30am	8/10 10:52pm	9/9 10:52am	10/8 9:42pm	11/7 7:52am	12/6 8:03pm	1/5/16 4:45am
6/30 10:43am	7/30 2:15am	8/28 5:24pm	9/27 7:34am	10/26 8:37pm	11/25 8:50am	12/24 8:31pm
7/19 3:00pm	8/17 6:21pm	9/16 10:27am	10/16 2:41am	11/14 6:28pm	12/14 9:17am	1/12/18 10:35pm
7/8 8:22am	8/6 8:29pm	9/5 10:43am	10/5 3:05am	11/3 9:01pm	12/3 3:19pm	1/2/19 8:24am
6/27 8:52pm	7/27* 5:22am	9/24 4:34am	10/23 8:39pm	11/22 3:19pm	12/22 10:55am	1/21/20 5:27am

Lunar Calendar 1920–1939

(Greenwich Mean Time/GMT)

		1st Tiger	2nd Hare	3rd Dragon	4th Snake	5th Horse
1920	*Monkey*	2/19 9:34pm	3/20 10:55am	4/18 9:43pm	5/18 6:25am	6/16 1:41pm
1921	*Cock*	2/8 12:36am	3/9 6:09pm	4/8 9:05am	5/7 9:01pm	6/6 6:14am
1922	*Dog*	1/27 11:48pm	2/26 6:47pm	3/28 1:03pm	4/27 5:03am	5/26* 6:04pm
1923	*Wild Boar*	2/15 7:07pm	3/17 12:51pm	4/16 6:28am	5/15 10:38pm	6/14 12:42pm
1924	*Rat*	2/5 1:38am	3/5 3:58pm	4/4 7:17am	5/3 11:00pm	6/2 2:34pm
1925	*Buffalo*	1/24 2:45pm	2/23 2:12am	3/24 2:03pm	4/23* 2:28am	6/21 6:17am
1926	*Tiger*	2/12 5:20pm	3/14 3:20am	4/12 12:56pm	5/11 10:55pm	6/10 10:08am
1927	*Hare*	2/2 8:19pm	3/3 7:24pm	4/2 4:24am	5/1 12:40pm	5/30 9:06pm
1928	*Dragon*	1/22 8:19pm	2/21* 9:41am	4/20 5:25am	5/19 1:14pm	6/17 8:42pm
1929	*Snake*	2/9 5:55pm	3/11 8:36am	4/9 8:32pm	5/9 6:07am	6/7 1:56pm
1930	*Horse*	1/29 7:07pm	2/28 1:33pm	3/30 5:46am	4/28 7:08pm	5/28 5:36am
1931	*Ram*	2/17 1:11pm	3/19 7:51am	4/18 1:00am	5/17 3:28pm	6/16 3:02pm
1932	*Monkey*	2/6 2:34pm	3/7 7:44am	4/6 1:21am	5/5 6:11pm	6/4 9:16am
1933	*Cock*	1/25 11:20pm	2/24 2:44pm	3/26 3:20am	4/24 6:38pm	5/24* 10:07am
1934	*Dog*	2/14 12:43am	3/15 12:08pm	4/13 11:57pm	5/13 12:30pm	6/12 2:11am
1935	*Wild Boar*	2/3 4:27pm	3/5 2:40am	4/3 12:11pm	5/2 9:36pm	6/1 7:52am
1936	*Rat*	1/24 8:18am	2/22 7:42pm	3/23* 5:14am	5/20 9:34pm	6/19 6:14am
1937	*Buffalo*	2/11 7:34am	3/12 7:32pm	4/11 5:10am	5/10 1:18pm	6/8 8:43pm
1938	*Tiger*	1/31 1:35pm	3/2 5:40am	3/31 6:52pm	4/30 5:28am	5/29 1:59pm
1939	*Hare*	2/19 8:28am	3/21 1:49am	4/19 4:35pm	5/19 4:25am	6/17 1:37pm

6th Ram	7th Monkey	8th Cock	9th Dog	10th Wild Boar	11th Rat	12th Buffalo
7/15 8:25pm	8/14 3:44am	9/12 12:51pm	10/12 12:50pm	11/10 4:05pm	12/10 10:04am	1/9/21 5:26am
7/5 1:36pm	8/3 8:17pm	9/2 3:33am	10/1 12:26pm	10/30 11:38pm	11/29 1:25pm	12/29 5:39a
7/24 12:47pm	8/22 8:34pm	9/21 6:38am	10/20 1:40pm	11/19 12:06am	12/18 12:20pm	1/17/23 2:41am
7/14 12:45pm	8/12 11:16am	9/10 8:52pm	10/10 6:05am	11/8 3:27pm	12/8 1:30am	1/6/24 12:48pm
7/2 5:35am	7/31 7:42pm	8/30 8:37am	9/28 8:16pm	10/28 6:57am	11/26 5:15pm	12/26 3:46am
7/20 10:40pm	8/19 1:14pm	9/18 4:12am	10/17 6:06pm	11/16 6:58am	12/15 7:05pm	1/14/26 6:35am
7/9 11:06pm	8/8 1:48pm	9/7 5:45am	10/6 10:13pm	11/5 2:34pm	12/5 6:11am	1/3/27 8:28pm
6/29 6:32am	7/28 5:36pm	8/27 6:45am	9/25 10:11pm	10/25 3:37pm	11/24 10:09am	12/24 4:13am
7/17 5:35am	8/15 2:48pm	9/14 2:20am	10/13 4:56pm	11/12 10:35am	12/12 6:06am	1/11/29 1:28am
7/6 8:47pm	8/5 3:40am	9/3 11:47Am	10/2 10:10pm	11/1 12:01pm	12/1 4:48am	12/30 11:42pm
6/26* 1:46pm	8/24 3:37am	9/22 11:42am	10/21 9:48pm	11/20 10:21am	12/20 1:24pm	1/18/31 6:35pm
7/15 12:20pm	8/13 8:27pm	9/12 4:26am	10/11 1:06pm	11/9 10:55pm	12/9 10:16am	1/7/32 11:29pm
7/3 10:20pm	8/2 9:42am	8/31 7:54pm	9/30 5:30am	10/29 2:56pm	11/28 12:43am	12/27 11:22am
7/22 4:03pm	8/21 5:48am	9/19 6:21pm	10/19 5:45am	11/17 4:24pm	12/17 2:53am	1/15/34 1:37pm
7/11 5:06pm	8/10 8:46am	9/9 12:20am	10/8 3:05pm	11/7 4:44am	12/6 5:25pm	1/5/35 5:20am
6/30 7:44pm	7/30 9:32am	8/29 1:00am	9/27 5:29pm	10/27 10:15am	11/26 2:36am	12/25 5:49pm
7/18 3:19pm	8/17 3:21am	9/15 5:41pm	10/15 10:20am	11/14 4:42am	12/13 11:25pm	1/12/37 4:47pm
7/8 4:13am	8/6 12:37pm	9/4 10:53pm	10/4 11:58am	11/3 4:16am	12/2 11:11pm	1/1/38 6:58pm
6/27 9:10pm	7/27* 3:53am	9/23 8:34pm	10/23 8:42am	11/22 12:05am	12/21 6:07pm	1/20/39 1:27pm
7/16 9:03pm	8/15 3:53am	9/13 11:22am	10/12 8:30pm	11/11 7:54am	12/10 9:45pm	1/9/40 1:53pm

Lunar Calendar 1940–1959

(Greenwich Mean Time/GMT)

		1st Tiger	2nd Hare	3rd Dragon	4th Snake	5th Horse
1940	*Dragon*	2/8 7:45am	3/9 2:23am	4/7 8:18pm	5/7 12:07pm	6/6 1:05am
1941	*Snake*	1/26 11:03pm	2/26 3:02am	3/27 8:14pm	4/26 1:23pm	5/26 5:18am
1942	*Horse*	2/15 10:03am	3/16 11:50pm	4/15 2:33pm	5/15 5:45am	6/13 9:02pm
1943	*Ram*	2/4 11:29pm	3/6 10:34am	4/4 9:43pm	5/4 9:43am	6/2 10:33pm
1944	*Monkey*	1/25 3:24	2/24 1:59am	3/24 11:36am	4/22* 8:43pm	6/20 5:00pm
1945	*Cock*	2/12 5:33pm	3/14 3:51am	4/12 12:30pm	5/11 8:21pm	6/10 4:26am
1946	*Dog*	2/2 4:43am	3/3 6:01pm	4/2 4:37am	5/1 1:16pm	5/30 8:49pm
1947	*Wild Boar*	1/22 8:34am	2/21* 2:00am	4/21 4:19am	5/20 1:44pm	6/18 9:26pm
1948	*Rat*	2/10 3:02am	3/10 9:15pm	4/9 1:17pm	5/9 2:30am	6/7 12:55pm
1949	*Buffalo*	1/29 2:42am	2/27 8:55pm	3/29 3:11pm	4/28 8:02am	5/27 10:24pm
1950	*Tiger*	2/16 10:53pm	3/18 3:20pm	4/17 8:25am	5/17 12:54am	6/15 3:53pm
1951	*Hare*	2/6 7:54am	3/7 8:51pm	4/6 10:52am	5/6 1:26am	6/4 4:40pm
1952	*Dragon*	1/26 10:26pm	2/25 9:16am	3/25 8:13pm	4/24 7:27am	5/23* 7:28pm
1953	*Snake*	2/14 1:10am	3/15 11:05am	4/13 8:09pm	5/13 5:06am	6/11 2:55pm
1954	*Horse*	2/3 3:55pm	3/5 3:11am	4/3 12:25pm	5/2 8:22pm	6/1 4:03am
1955	*Ram*	1/24 1:07am	2/22 3:54pm	3/24* 3:42am	5/21 8:59pm	6/20 4:12am
1956	*Monkey*	2/11 9:38pm	3/12 1:37pm	4/11 2:39am	5/10 1:04pm	6/8 9:29pm
1957	*Cock*	1/30 9:25pm	3/1 4:12pm	3/31 9:19am	4/30 11:54am	5/28 11:39am
1958	*Dog*	2/18 3:38pm	3/20 9:50am	4/19 3:23am	5/18 7:00pm	6/17 7:59am
1959	*Wild Boar*	7/2 7:22pm	3/9 10:51am	4/8 3:29am	5/7 8:11pm	6/6 11:53am

6th Ram	7th Monkey	8th Cock	9th Dog	10th Wild Boar	11th Rat	12th Buffalo
7/4 11:28am	8/3 8:09pm	9/2 4:15am	10/1 12:41pm	10/30 10:03pm	11/29 8:42am	12/28 8:56pm
6/24* 7:22pm	8/22 6:34pm	9/21 4:38am	10/20 2:20pm	11/19 12:04am	12/18 10:18am	1/16/42 9:2pm
8/12 12:03pm	9/10 2:28am	10/10 3:53pm	11/8 4:06am	12/8 3:19pm	1/6/43 1:59am	7/13 12:38pm
7/2 12:44pm	8/1 4:06am	8/30 7:59pm	9/29 11:29am	10/29 1:59am	11/27 3:23am	12/27 3:50am
7/20 5:42am	8/18 8:25pm	9/17 12:37pm	10/17 5:35am	11/15 10:29pm	12/15 2:35pm	1/14/45 5:07am
7/9 1:35pm	8/8 12:32am	9/6 1:44pm	10/6 5:22am	11/4 11:11pm	12/4 6:07pm	1/3/46 12:30pm
6/29 4:06am	7/27 11:54am	8/26 9:07pm	9/25 8:45am	10/24 11:32pm	11/23 5:24pm	12/23 1:06pm
7/18 4:15am	8/16 11:12am	9/14 7:28pm	10/14 6:10am	11/12 8:01pm	12/12 12:53pm	1/11/48 7:45am
7/6 9:09pm	8/5 4:13am	9/3 11:21am	10/2 7:42pm	11/1 6:03am	11/30 6:44pm	12/30 9:45am
6/26 10:02am	7/25* 7:33pm	9/22 12:21pm	10/21 9:23pm	11/20 7:29am	12/19 6:56pm	1/18/50 9:00am
7/15 5:05am	8/13 4:48pm	9/12 3:29am	10/11 1:33pm	11/9 11:25pm	12/9 9:29am	1/7/51 8:10pm
7/4 7:48am	8/2 10:39pm	9/1 12:50pm	10/1 1:57am	10/30 1:54pm	11/29 1:00am	12/27 11:43am
7/22 12:31am	8/20 4:20pm	9/19 8:22am	10/18 12:42pm	11/17 1:56pm	12/17 3:02am	1/15/53 3:08pm
7/11 2:28am	8/9 4:10pm	9/8 7:48am	10/8 12:40am	6/11 5:58pm	12/6 10:48am	1/5/54 2:21am
6/30 12:26pm	7/29 10:20pm	8/28 10:21am	9/27 12:50am	10/26 5:47pm	11/25 12:30pm	12/25 7:33am
7/19 11:35am	8/17 7:58pm	9/16 6:19am	10/15 7:32pm	11/14 12:02pm	12/14 7:07am	1/13/56 3:01am
7/8 4:38am	8/6 11:25am	9/4 6:57pm	10/4 4:25am	11/2 4:44pm	12/2 8:13am	1/1/57 2:14am
6/27 8:53pm	7/27 4:28am	8/25* 11:33am	10/23 4:43am	11/21 4:19pm	12/21 6:12am	1/19/58 10:08pm
7/16 7:33pm	8/15 4:33am	9/13 1:02pm	10/12 9:52pm	11/11 7:34am	12/10 6:23pm	1/9/59 6:34am
7/6 2:00am	8/4 2:34pm	9/3 1:56am	10/2 12:31pm	10/31 10:41pm	11/30 8:46am	12/29 7:09pm

Lunar Calendar 1960–1979

(Greenwich Mean Time/GMT)

		1st Tiger	2nd Hare	3rd Dragon	4th Snake	5th Horse
1960	*Rat*	1/28 6:15am	2/26 6:24am	3/27 7:37am	4/25 9:44pm	5/25 12:26pm
1961	*Buffalo*	2/15 8:10am	3/16 6:51pm	4/15 5:37am	5/14 4:54pm	6/13 5:16am
1962	*Tiger*	2/5 12:10am	3/6 10:31am	4/4 7:45pm	5/4 4:25am	6/2 1:27pm
1963	*Hare*	1/25 1:42pm	2/24 2:06am	3/25 12:10pm	4/23* 8:29pm	6/21 11:46am
1964	*Dragon*	2/13 1:01pm	3/14 2:14am	4/12 12:37pm	5/11 9:02pm	6/10 4:22am
1965	*Snake*	2/1 4:36pm	3/3 9:56am	4/2 12:21am	5/1 11:56am	5/30 9:12pm
1966	*Horse*	1/21 3:46pm	2/20 10:49am	3/22* 4:46am	5/20 9:42am	6/18 8:09pm
1967	*Ram*	2/9 10:44am	3/11 4:30am	4/9 10:20pm	5/9 2:55pm	6/8 5:13am
1968	*Monkey*	1/29 5:29pm	2/28 7:56am	3/28 11:48pm	4/27 4:21pm	5/27 8:30am
1969	*Cock*	2/16 4:25pm	3/18 4:51am	4/16 6:16pm	5/16 8:26am	6/14 11:09pm
1970	*Dog*	2/6 7:13am	3/7 5:42pm	4/6 4:09am	5/5 2:51pm	6/4 2:21am
1971	*Wild Boar*	1/26 10:55pm	2/25 9:49am	3/26 7:23pm	4/25 4:02am	5/24* 12:32pm
1972	*Rat*	2/15 12:29am	3/15 11:35am	4/13 8:31pm	5/13 4:08am	6/10 11:30am
1973	*Buffalo*	2/3 10:23am	5/3 1:07am	4/3 12:45pm	5/2 9:55pm	6/1 5:35am
1974	*Tiger*	1/23 11:02am	2/22 5:34am	3/23 9:24pm	4/22* 10:16am	6/20 4:56am
1975	*Hare*	2/11 5:17am	3/12 11:47pm	4/11 4:39pm	5/11 7:05am	6/9 6:49pm
1976	*Dragon*	1/31 6:20am	2/28 11:25pm	3/30 5:08pm	4/29 10:19am	5/29 1:47am
1977	*Snake*	2/18 3:37am	3/19 6:33pm	4/18 10:35am	5/18 2:51am	6/16 6:23pm
1978	*Horse*	2/7 2:54pm	3/9 2:36am	4/7 3:15pm	5/7 4:47am	6/5 7:01pm
1979	*Ram*	1/28 6:20am	2/26 4:45pm	3/28 3:00am	4/26 1:15pm	5/25 12:00pm

6th Ram	7th Monkey	8th Cock	9th Dog	10th Wild Boar	11th Rat	12th Buffalo
6/24* 3:27am	8/22 9:15am	9/20 11:12pm	10/20 12:02pm	11/18 11:46pm	12/18 10:47am	1/16/61 9:30pm
7/12 7:11pm	8/11 10:36am	9/10 2:50am	10/9 6:52pm	11/8 9:58am	12/7 11:52pm	1/6/62 12:35pm
7/1 11:52pm	7/31 12:24pm	8/30 3:09am	9/28 7:39pm	10/28 1:05pm	11/27 6:29am	12/26 10:59pm
7/20 8:43pm	8/19 7:35am	9/17 8:51pm	10/17 12:43am	11/16 6:50am	12/16 2:06am	1/14/64 8:43pm
7/9 11:31am	8/7 7:17pm	9/6 4:34am	10/5 4:20pm	11/4 7:16am	12/4 1:18am	1/2/65 9:07pm
6/29 4:52am	7/28 11:45am	8/26 6:50pm	9/25 3:18am	10/24 2:11pm	11/23 4:10am	12/22 9:03pm
7/18 4:30am	8/16 11:48am	9/14 7:13pm	10/14 3:52am	11/12 2:26pm	12/12 3:13am	1/10/67 6:06pm
7/7 5:00pm	8/6 2:48am	9/4 11:37am	10/3 8:24pm	11/2 5:48am	12/1 4:10pm	12/31 3:38am
6/25 10:24pm	7/25* 11:49am	9/21 11:08pm	10/21 9:44pm	11/20 8:01am	12/19 6:19pm	1/18/69 4:59am
7/14 2:11pm	8/13 5:16am	9/11 7:56am	10/11 9:39am	11/9 10:11pm	12/9 9:42am	1/7/70 8:35pm
7/3 3:18pm	8/2 5:58am	8/31 10:01pm	9/30 2:31pm	10/30 6:28am	11/28 9:14pm	12/28 10:43am
7/22 9:15am	8/20 10:53pm	9/19 2:42pm	10/19 7:59am	11/18 1:46am	12/17 7:03pm	1/16/72 10:52am
7/10 7:39pm	8/9 5:26am	9/7 5:28pm	10/7 8:08am	11/6 1:21am	12/6 8:24pm	1/4/73 3:42pm
6/30 11:39am	7/29 6:59pm	8/28 3:25am	9/26 1:54pm	10/26 3:17am	11/24 7:55pm	12/24 3:07pm
7/19 12:06pm	8/17 7:02pm	9/16 2:45am	10/15 12:25pm	11/14 12:53am	12/13 4:25pm	1/12/75 10:20am
7/9 4:10am	8/7 11:57am	9/5 7:19pm	10/5 3:23am	11/3 1:05pm	12/3 12:50am	1/1/76 2:40pm
6/27 2:50pm	7/27 1:39am	8/25* 11:01am	10/23 5:10am	11/21 3:11pm	12/21 2:08am	1/19/77 2:11pm
7/16 8:36am	8/14 9:31pm	9/13 9:23am	10/12 8:31pm	11/11 7:09am	12/10 5:33pm	1/9/78 4:00am
7/5 9:50am	8/4 1:01am	9/2 4:09pm	10/2 6:41am	10/31 8:06am	11/30 8:19am	12/29 7:36pm
6/24* 11:58am	8/22 5:10pm	9/21 9:47am	10/21 2:23am	11/19 8:04pm	12/19 8:23am	1/17/80 9:19pm

Lunar Calendar 1980–1999

(Greenwich Mean Time/GMT)

		1st Tiger	2nd Hare	3rd Dragon	4th Snake	5th Horse
1980	*Monkey*	2/16 8:51am	3/16 6:56pm	4/15 3:46am	5/14 12:00am	6/12 8:38pm
1981	*Cock*	2/4 10:14pm	3/6 10:31am	4/4 8:19pm	5/4 4:19am	6/2 11:32am
1982	*Dog*	1/25 4:56am	2/23 9:13pm	3/25 10:17am	4/23* 8:29pm	6/21 11:52am
1983	*Wild Boar*	2/13 12:32am	3/14 5:43pm	4/13 7:58am	5/12 7:25pm	6/11 4:37am
1984	*Rat*	2/1 11:46pm	3/2 6:31pm	4/1 12:10pm	5/1 3:45am	5/30 4:48pm
1985	*Buffalo*	2/19 6:43pm	3/21 11:59am	4/20 5:22am	5/19 9:41pm	6/18 11:58am
1986	*Tiger*	2/9 12:55am	3/10 2:52pm	4/9 6:08am	5/8 10:10pm	6/7 2:00pm
1987	*Hare*	1/29 1:45pm	2/28 12:51am	3/29 12:46pm	4/28 1:34am	5/27 3:13pm
1988	*Dragon*	2/17 3:54pm	3/18 2:02am	4/16 12:00am	5/15 10:11pm	6/14 9:14am
1989	*Snake*	2/6 7:37am	3/7 6:19pm	4/6 3:33am	5/5 11:46am	6/3 7:53pm
1990	*Horse*	1/26 7:20pm	2/25 8:54am	3/26 7:48pm	4/25 4:27am	5/24* 11:47am
1991	*Ram*	2/14 5:32pm	3/16 8:10am	4/14 7:38pm	5/14 4:36am	6/12 12:06pm
1992	*Monkey*	2/3 7:00pm	3/4 1:22pm	4/3 5:01am	5/2 5:44pm	6/1 3:57am
1993	*Cock*	1/22 6:27pm	2/21 1:05pm	3/23* 7:14am	5/21 2:07pm	6/20 1:52am
1994	*Dog*	2/10 2:30pm	3/12 7:05am	4/11 12:17am	5/10 5:07pm	6/9 8:26am
1995	*Wild Boar*	1/30 10:48pm	3/1 11:48am	3/31 2:09am	4/29 5:36pm	5/29 9:27am
1996	*Rat*	2/18 11:30pm	3/19 10:45am	4/17 10:49pm	5/17 11:46am	6/16 1:26am
1997	*Buffalo*	2/7 3:06pm	3/9 1:15am	4/7 11:02am	5/6 8:47pm	6/5 7:04am
1998	*Tiger*	1/28 6:01am	2/26 5:26am	3/28 3:14am	4/26 11:41am	5/25* 7:32pm
1999	*Hare*	2/16 6:39am	3/17 6:48pm	4/16 4:22am	5/15 12:05pm	6/13 7:03pm

6th Ram	7th Monkey	8th Cock	9th Dog	10th Wild Boar	11th Rat	12th Buffalo
7/12 6:46am	8/10 7:09pm	9/9 10:00am	10/9 2:50am	11/7 8:43pm	12/7 2:35pm	1/6/81 7:24am
7/1 7:03am	7/31 3:52am	8/29 2:43pm	9/28 4:07am	10/27 8:13pm	11/26 2:38pm	12/26 10:10am
7/20 6:57pm	8/19 2:45am	9/17 12:09pm	10/17 12:04am	11/15 3:10pm	12/15 9:18am	1/14/83 5:08am
7/10 12:18pm	8/8 7:18pm	9/7 2:35am	10/6 11:16am	11/4 10:21pm	12/4 12:26pm	1/3/84 5:16am
6/29 3:18am	7/28 11:51am	8/26 7:25pm	9/25 3:11am	10/24* 12:08pm	12/22 11:47am	1/21/85 2:28am
7/17 11:56pm	8/16 10:05am	9/14 7:20pm	10/14 4:33am	11/12 2:20pm	12/12 12:54am	1/10/86 12:22pm
7/7 4:55am	8/5 6:36pm	9/4 7:10am	10/3 6:55pm	11/2 6:02am	12/1 4:43pm	12/31 3:10am
6/26* 5:37am	8/24 11:59am	9/23 3:08am	10/22 5:28pm	11/21 6:33am	12/20 6:25pm	1/19/88 5:26am
7/13 9:53pm	8/12 12:31pm	9/11 4:49am	10/10 9:49pm	11/9 2:20pm	12/9 5:36am	1/7/89 7:22pm
7/3 5:59am	8/1 5:06pm	8/31 6:45am	9/29 10:47pm	10/29 4:27pm	11/28 10:41am	12/28 4:20am
7/22 2:54am	8/20 12:39pm	9/19 12:46am	10/18 3:37pm	11/17 9:05am	12/17 4:22am	1/15/91 11:50pm
7/12 7:06pm	8/10 2:28am	9/8 11:01am	10/7 9:39pm	11/6 11:11am	12/6 3:56am	1/4/92 11:10pm
6/30 12:18pm	7/29 7:35pm	8/28 2:42am	9/26 10:40am	10/25 8:34pm	11/24 9:11am	12/24 12:43am
7/19 11:24am	8/17 7:28pm	9/16 3:10am	10/15 11:36am	11/13 9:34pm	12/13 9:27am	1/11/94 11:10pm
7/8 9:37pm	8/7 8:45am	9/5 6:33pm	10/5 3:55am	11/3 1:35pm	12/2 11:54pm	1/1/95 10:56am
6/28 12:50am	7/27 3:13pm	8/26* 4:31am	10/24 4:36am	11/22 3:43pm	12/22 2:22am	1/20/96 12:51pm
7/15 4:15pm	8/14 7:34am	9/12 11:07pm	10/12 2:14pm	11/11 4:16am	12/10 4:56pm	1/9/97 4:26am
7/4 6:40pm	8/3 8:14am	9/1 11:52pm	10/1 4:52pm	10/31 10:01am	11/30 2:14am	12/29 4:57pm
7/23 1:44pm	8/22 2:03am	9/20 5:02pm	10/20 10:09am	11/19 4:27am	12/18 10:42pm	1/17/99 3:46pm
7/13 2:24am	8/11 11:09am	9/9 10:02pm	10/9 11:34am	11/8 3:53am	12/7 10:32pm	1/6/00 6:14pm

Lunar Calendar 2000–2019

(Greenwich Mean Time/GMT)

		1st Tiger	2nd Hare	3rd Dragon	4th Snake	5th Horse
2000	*Dragon*	2/5 1:03pm	3/6 5:17am	4/4 6:12pm	5/4 4:12am	6/2 12:14pm
2001	*Snake*	1/24 1:07pm	2/23 8:21am	3/25 1:21am	4/23* 3:26pm	6/21 11:58am
2002	*Horse*	2/12 7:41am	3/14 2:03am	4/12 7:21pm	5/12 10:45am	6/10 11:47pm
2003	Ram	2/1 10:48am	3/3 2:35am	4/1 7:19pm	5/1 12:15pm	5/31 4:20am
2004	*Monkey*	1/21 9:05pm	2/20* 9:18am	4/19 1:21pm	5/19 4:52am	6/17 8:27pm
2005	*Cock*	2/8 10:38pm	3/10 9:10am	4/8 8:32pm	5/8 8:46am	6/6 9:55pm
2006	*Dog*	1/29 2:15pm	2/28 12:31pm	3/29 10:15am	4/27 7:44pm	5/27 5:26am
2007	*Wild Boar*	2/17 4:14pm	3/19 2:43am	4/17 11:36am	5/16 7:27pm	6/15 3:13am
2008	*Rat*	2/7 3:45am	3/7 5:14pm	4/6 3:55am	5/5 12:18pm	6/3 7:23pm
2009	*Buffalo*	1/26 7:55am	2/25 1:35am	3/26 4:06pm	4/25 3:23am	5/24* 12:11pm
2010	*Tiger*	2/14 2:51am	3/15 9:01pm	4/14 12:20pm	5/14 1:04am	6/12 11:15am
2011	*Hare*	2/3 2:31am	3/4 8:46pm	4/3 2:32pm	5/3 6:51am	6/1 9:03pm
2012	*Dragon*	1/23 7:39am	2/21 10:35pm	3/22 2:37pm	4/21* 7:19am	6/19 3:02pm
2013	*Snake*	2/10 7:20am	3/11 7:51pm	4/10 9:35am	5/10 12:29am	6/8 3:56pm
2014	*Horse*	1/30 9:39pm	3/1 8:00am	3/30 6:45pm	4/29 6:14am	5/28 6:40pm
2015	*Ram*	2/18 11:47pm	3/20 9:36am	4/18 6:57pm	5/18 4:13am	6/16 2:05pm
2016	*Monkey*	2/8 2:39pm	3/9 1:55am	4/7 11:24am	5/6 7:30am	6/5 3:00am
2017	*Cock*	1/28 12:07am	2/26 2:59pm	3/28 2:57am	4/26 12:16pm	5/25 7:45pm
2018	*Dog*	2/15 9:05pm	3/17 1:12pm	4/16 1:57am	5/15 11:48am	6/13 7:43pm
2019	*Wild Boar*	2/4 9:04pm	3/6 4:04pm	4/5 8:51am	5/4 10:46pm	6/3 10:02am

6th Ram	7th Monkey	8th Cock	9th Dog	10th Wild Boar	11th Rat	12th Buffalo
7/1 7:20pm	7/31 2:25am	8/29 10:19am	9/27 7:53pm	10/27 7:58am	11/25 11:11pm	12/25 5:22pm
7/20 7:44pm	8/19 2:55am	9/17 3:10am	10/6 11:18am	11/4 8:35pm	12/4 7:34am	1/2/03 8:23pm
7/10 10:26am	8/8 7:15pm	9/7 3:10am	10/6 11:18am	11/4 8:35pm	12/4 7:34am	1/2/03 8:23pm
6/29 6:39pm	7/29 6:53am	8/27 5:26pm	9/26 3:09am	10/25 12:50pm	11/23 10:59pm	12/23 11:43am
7/17 11:24am	8/16 1:24am	9/14 2:29pm	10/14 2:48am	11/12 2:27pm	12/12 1:29am	1/10/05 12:03pm
7/6 12:03pm	8/5 3:05am	9/3 6:45pm	10/3 10:28am	11/2 1:25am	12/1 3:01pm	12/31 3:12am
6:26 4:05pm	7/25* 4:31am	9/22 11:45am	10/22 5:14am	11/20 10:18pm	12/20 2:01pm	1/19/07 4:01am
7/14 12:04pm	8/12 11:03pm	9/11 12:44pm	10/11 5:01am	11/9 11:03pm	12/9 5:40pm	1/8/08 11:37am
7/3 3:19am	8/1 11:13am	8/30 8:58pm	9/29 9:12am	10/29 12:14am	11/27 5:55pm	12/27 1:22pm
7/22 2:35am	8/20 10:02am	9/18 6:44pm	10/18 5:33am	11/16 7:14pm	12/16 12:02pm	1/15/10 7:11am
7/11 7:41pm	8/10 3:08am	9/8 10:30am	10/7 6:45pm	11/6 4:52am	12/5 5:36pm	1/4/11 9:03am
7/1 8:54am	7/30 6:40pm	8/29 3:04am	9/27 11:09am	10/26 7:56pm	11/25 6:10am	12/24 6:06pm
7/19 4:24am	8/17 3:55pm	9/16 2:11am	10/15 12:03pm	11/13 10:08pm	12/13 8:42am	1/11/13 7:44pm
7/8 7:14am	8/6 9:51pm	9/5 11:36am	10/5 12:35am	11/3 12:50pm	12/3 12:22am	1/1/14 11:14am
6/27 8:09am	7/26 10:42pm	8/25 2:13pm	9/24* 6:14am	11/22 12:32pm	12/22 1:36am	1/20/15 1:14pm
7/16 1:24am	8/14 2:54pm	9/13 6:41am	10/13 12:06am	11/11 5:47pm	12/11 10:30am	1/10/16 1:31am
7/4 11:01am	8/2 8:45pm	9/1 9:03am	10/1 12:12am	10/30 5:38pm	11/29 12:18pm	12/29 6:53am
6/24* 2:31am	8/21 6:30pm	9/20 5:30am	10/19 7:12pm	11/18 11:42am	12/18 6:31am	1/17/18 2:17am
7/13 2:48am	8/11 9:58am	9/9 6:02pm	10/9 3:47am	11/7 4:02pm	12/7 7:20am	1/6/19 1:28pm
7/2 7:16pm	8/1 3:12am	8/30 10:37am	9/28 6:26pm	10/28 3:39am	11/26 3:06pm	12/26 5:13am

Lunar Calendar 2020–2025

(Greenwich Mean Time/GMT)

		1st Tiger	2nd Hare	3rd Dragon	4th Snake	5th Horse
2020	*Rat*	1/24 9:42pm	2/23 3:32pm	3/24 9:28am	4/23* 2:26am	6/21 6:42am
2021	*Buffalo*	2/11 7:06pm	3/13 10:21am	4/12 2:31am	5/11 7:00pm	6/10 10:53am
2022	*Tiger*	2/1 5:46am	3/2 5:35pm	4/1 6:25am	4/30 8:28pm	5/30 11:30am
2023	*Hare*	1/21 8:53pm	2/20* 7:06am	4/20 4:13am	5/19 3:53pm	6/18 4:37am
2024	*Dragon*	2/9 10:59pm	3/10 9:01am	4/8 6:21pm	5/8 3:22am	6/6 12:38pm
2025	*Snake*	1/29 12:36pm	2/28 12:45am	3/29 10:58am	4/27 7:31pm	5/27 3:02am

Chart to Copy

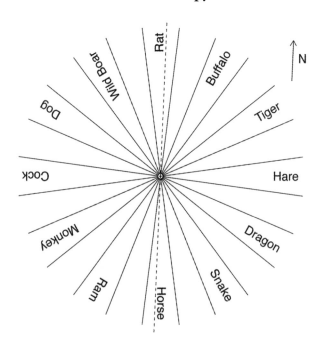

The Twelve Animal Signs and Their Sectors

6th Ram	7th Monkey	8th Cock	9th Dog	10th Wild Boar	11th Rat	12th Buffalo
7/20 5:33pm	8/19 2:42am	9/17 11:00am	10/16 9:31pm	11/15 5:07am	12/14 4:17pm	1/13/21 5:00am
7/10 1:17am	8/8 1:50pm	9/7 12:52am	10/6 11:06am	4/11 9:15pm	12/4 7:43am	1/2/22 6:34pm
6/29 3:52am	7/28 6:55pm	8/27 9:17am	9/25 10:55pm	10/25 11:49am	11/23 11:57pm	12/23 11:17am
7/17 6:32pm	8/16 9:38am	9/15 1:40am	10/14 5:55pm	11/13 9:28am	12/12 11:32pm	1/11/24 11:58am
7/5 10:58pm	8/4 11:13am	9/3 1:56am	10/2 6:49pm	11/1 12:47pm	12/1 6:22am	12/30 10:27pm
6/25* 10:32am	8/23 6:07am	9/21 7:54pm	10/21 12:25pm	11/20 6:47am	12/20 1:43am	1/18/26 7:52pm

Chart to Copy

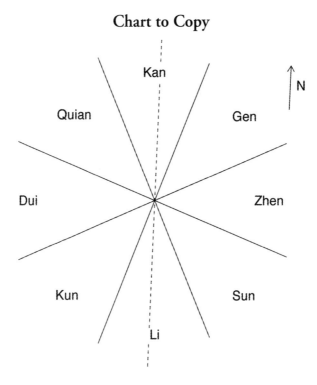

The Eight Trigrams and Their Sectors

The Authors

Wilhelm Gerstung, born in 1948, has worked as a feng shui consultant and feng shui trainer for many years. He has been actively involved with feng shui in theory and practice since the beginning of the 1980s. Within this context, he has long been interested in the subtle energies of the sleeping environment. His particular focus has been fundamental correlations between very specific health disorders and location-dependent disruptive energetic fields.

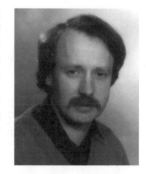

Jens Mehlhase, born in 1956, is an internist and has been a feng shui consultant for many years. Even during his studies, he was intensively involved in methods of alternative healing. In the process, he also learned about Western methods of examining the sleeping area using the pendulum or dowser. Combining this knowledge with the Eastern knowledge of feng Shui particularly fascinated him since he also found an extensive system for evaluating the quality of space and time.

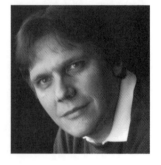

Wilhelm Gerstung and Jens Mehlhase have worked together as a team for many years. They have developed a system for evaluating the direction of the individual energies of feng shui and have dedicated themselves to mutually researching and differentiating a great variety of subtle energy forms. In addition to the development of their own theoretical concepts, one major focus of their work has been the development of new feng shui remedies. Both have been leading seminars on the topic of feng shui for years and have trained many feng shui consultants. In addition to this current volume, the following books by the two authors have been published in Germany: *Das grosse Feng Shui Haus- und Wohnungsbuch* (1998) and *Das grosse Feng Shui Garten- und Pflanzenbuch* (2000).

Expression of Thanks

We would like to thank Susi Keidel-Gerstung, Wilhelm Gerstung's wife, for the long years of support in our feng shui research and turning this book project into reality.

We would also like to thank Mr. Hoenel (Kerzell/Germany) for the concrete technical realization of some of our feng shui ideas into reality.

Information and Advice

Most of the feng shui products, like Feng Shui Power Disc 99 (invented by the authors), tensors (single-handed dowsers), L-shaped dowsing rods, WS Frequency Devices, cork tiles of a suitable quality, as well as other feng shui remedies are available in various shops and mailing-catalogs.

For Tachyonized Silica Discs contact:
www.tachyon-energy.com

For the Feng Shui Power Disc 99. (Wholesale and Retail) contact:
Website: www.fengshui-newengland.com
Email: wernerbrandmaier@yahoo.com
Toll free: 877-752-7888
Fax: 207-772-8188

If you want to write to Werner Brandmaier, use the following address:
Feng Shui of New England
Werner Brandmaier, 193 Concord Street
Portland, Maine 04103, USA
Tel. 207-772-7888
Werner Brandmaier is trained by the authors. He also gives information about business and home consultations, offers seminars and trainings.

More information under:
e-mail: wgerstung@feng-shui-kanyu.com
www.feng-shui-kanyu.com
Phone (++49-551) 91006
Fax (++49-551) 91008

You can write to the authors using the following address:
Institut fuer angewandtes Kanyu, Lotzestr. 3, D-37083 Goettingen, Germany

Herbs and other natural health products and information are often available at natural food stores or metaphysical bookstores. If you cannot find what you need locally, you can contact one of the following sources of supply.

Sources of Supply:

The following companies have an extensive selection of useful products and a long track-record of fulfillment. They have natural body care, aromatherapy, flower essences, crystals and tumbled stones, homeopathy, herbal products, vitamins and supplements, videos, books, audio tapes, candles, incense and bulk herbs, teas, massage tools and products and numerous alternative health items across a wide range of categories.

WHOLESALE:

Wholesale suppliers sell to stores and practitioners, not to individual consumers buying for their own personal use. Individual consumers should contact the RETAIL supplier listed below. Wholesale accounts should contact with business name, resale number or practitioner license in order to obtain a wholesale catalog and set up an account.

Lotus Light Enterprises, Inc.

P. O. Box 1008
Silver Lake, WI 531 70 USA
262 889 8501 (phone)
262 889 8591 (fax)
800 548 3824 (toll free order line)

RETAIL:

Retail suppliers provide products by mail order direct to consumers for their personal use. Stores or practitioners should contact the wholesale supplier listed above.

Internatural

33719 116th Street
Twin Lakes, WI 53181 USA
800 643 4221 (toll free order line)
262 889 8581 office phone
WEB SITE: www.internatural.com

Web site includes an extensive annotated catalog of more than 7000 products that can be ordered "on line" for your convenience 24 hours a day, 7 days a week.

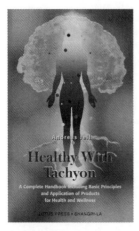

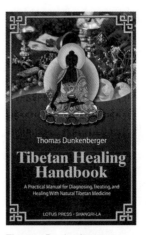

Andreas Jell

Healthy with Tachyon

A Complete Handbook Including Basic Principles and Application of Products for Health and Wellness

The comprehensive handbook for using tachyonized materials. A completely new chapter of human history has begun with the possibility of directly applying tachyon energy for healing and development.

Today, you can directly strengthen your powers of self-healing by using tachyonized materials. These powers will then organize perfect healing and development (anti-entropy) through their own dynamic.

Andreas Jell presents the details of all the currently available tachyonized products, as well as how they can be best applied. A brief introduction to the theoretic basis, reports on experiences by users, background knowledge from the fields of medicine and biology, and topics related to the use of tachyon energy provide a comprehensive look at this new, fascinating spiritual/scientific technology.

144 pages · $12.95
ISBN 0-914955-58-6

Thomas Dunkenberger

Tibetan Healing Handbook

A Practical Manual for Diagnosing, Treating, and Healing with Natural Tibetan Medicine

An introduction to one of the oldest healing systems
Tibetan Natural Medicine - Comprehensive and Easy to Understand
This book will inform you about the essential correlations and approaches taken by the Tibetan science of healing.
It describes the entire spectrum of application possibilities for those who want to study Tibetan medicine and use it for treatment purposes. At the same time, it provides information about holistic remedies so that interested readers can take action to restore their inner harmony and health. *Tibetan Healing Handbook* discusses the fundamental principles of health and causes of disease. These include non-visible forces and biorhythmic-planetary influences; classic Tibetan forms of diagnosis, the foremost of which are pulse and urine examination; advice on behavior and healing approaches to dietary habits, as well as the accessory therapeutic possibilities of oil massages, moxabustion, hydrotherapy, humoral excretion procedures, and much more. The famous Tibetan remedies are described in detail.

240 pages · $15.95
ISBN 0-914955-66-7

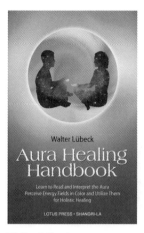

Walter Lübeck

Aura Healing Handbook

Learn to Read and Interpret the Aura · Perceive Energy Fields in Color and Utilize Them for Holistic Healing

Anyone can basically learn to see auras. Walter Lübeck's Aura Healing Handbook is a step-by-step instruction manual: By increasing your sensitivity for subtle vibrations, it will ultimately lead you into the fascinating world of seeing auras.

The author explains how to develop your "psychic" powers. He describes the different ways in which you can use these powers and the areas to which you can apply them. As a result, you can see subtle energies and they will reveal their secrets to you.

Aura reading serves as a diagnostic aid in recognizing health disorders long before they manifest themselves within the body in the form of pain or unwellness. Reading the aura is the first step to healing your energies and emotions in the subtle realm.

224 pages · $15.95
ISBN 0-914955-61-6

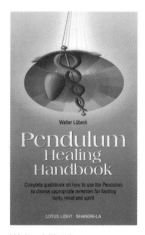

Walter Lübeck

Pendulum Healing Handbook

Complete Guidebook on How to Use the Pendulum to Choose Appropriate Remedies for Healing Body, Mind and Spirit.

If you want to learn every aspect of how to use a pendulum, particularly in relation to methods of alternative healing, this book is for you.

This book contains many of the most important pendulum tables from the areas of nutrition, aromas, Bach Flowers, gemstones, chakras, herbs, relationships, etc., and shows how to use them, along with the limits of their application. Walter Lübeck begins with the selection of the right pendulum, shows the correct way to hold it, and also explains the possibilities of energetic cleansing. With 125 pendulum tables.

208 pages · $15.95
ISBN 0-914955-54-3

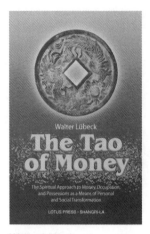

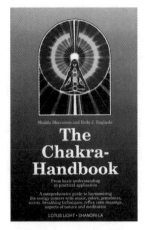

Walter Lübeck

The Tao of Money

The Spiritual Approach to Money, Occupation, and Possessions as a Means of Personal and Social Transformation

The Tao of Money explores how to heal material consciousness. For author Walter Lübeck, money can be equated with energy, something that manifests itself in every conceivable manner. This fascinating book about money contains many exercises on its spiritual meaning, work, occupation, and much more. How you treat money in your everyday life also expresses the inner state of your soul.

To a large extent, money has a deep spiritual dimension: Money activates the root chakra, wealth sets the love-of-life chakra into motion, and work affects the power chakra and the heart chakra. You can awaken the expression chakra through your job and use possessions to increase your kundalini energy. Discover what type of money person you are.

160 pages · $14.95
ISBN 0-914955-62-4

Shalila Sharamon and Bodo J. Baginski

The Chakra Handbook

From Basic Understanding to Practical Application

Knowledge of the energy centers provides us with deep, comprehensive insight into the effects the subtle powers have on the human organism. This book vividly describes the functioning of the energy centers. For practical work with the chakras this book offers a wealth of possibilities: the use of sounds, colors, gemstones, and fragrances with their own specific effects, augmented by meditation, breathing techniques, foot reflexology massage of the chakra points, and the instilling of universal life energy. The description of nature experiences, yoga practices, and the relationship of each indiviual chakra to the zodiac additionally provides inspiring and valuable insight.

192 pages · $14.95
ISBN 0-941524-85-X

For more information about natural health products see Sources of Supply on page 245.